Effective Clinical Supervision

Effective Clinical Supervision

edited by

Tony Ghaye and Sue Lillyman

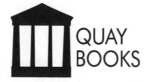

QUAY
BOOKS

Quay Books Division, MA Healthcare Ltd, St Jude's Church, Dulwich Road, London SE24 0PB

British Library Cataloguing-in-Publication Data
A catalogue record is available for this book

1st edition published May 2000
2nd edition published May 2007

© MA Healthcare Limited 2007
ISBN-10: 1-85642-332-8
ISBN-13: 978-185642-332-8

Printed in the UK by Athenaeum Press Ltd, Dukesway, Team Valley, Gateshead, NE11 0PZ

Contents

List of contributors

Tony Ghaye Cert Ed, B Ed(Hons) MA(Ed) PhD.
Chief Executive Officer of the Institute of Reflective Practice, UK; Professor in Educare; Visiting Professor at the University of Luleå, Sweden, and Senior International Consultant at the Beijing-Geely University, China.

Tony Ghaye is is founder and Editor-in-Chief of the peer-reviewed journal *Reflective Practice*. He has an international reputation in enabling individuals, work teams and whole organisations to increase performance through appreciative and strengths-based reflective learning. His most recent books include *Developing the Reflective Healthcare Team* and *Building the Reflective Healthcare Organisation* published by Blackwell Publishing, Oxford. Tony is interested in using experienced-based reflective learning to build and sustain responsive services and to support those in human service work so that they may act ethically and with moral courage.

Karen Latimer RGN, MSc, BA, Dip in Counselling
Senior Lecturer at the Institute of Health, Social Care and Psychology, University of Worcester.

Karen Latimer began her nursing career in 1981 at East Birmingham Hospital, West Midlands. She then worked within adult acute settings before making the transition to nurse education in 1999. Her role as a professional development nurse at Birmingham Heartlands Hospital (formally East Birmingham Hospital) involved teaching and developing educational programmes for all grades of nurses. It was during this time that she became involved in clinical supervision and was involved in a joint venture between three other West Midlands trusts in an open learning package called 'Super vision'. Karen also became a member of the West Midlands regional strategy group for clinical supervision.

Her current position as a senior lecturer at the University of Worcester involves being a module co-ordinator on the pre-registration diploma in higher education and degree course nurse training programmes. Karen is also currently involved in supporting Worcestershire Acute Trust with the development of their strategy and clinical supervision workshops for supervisors.

Sue Lillyman MA, BSc(Nursing), RN, RM, DPSN, PGCE (FAHE).
Senior Lecturer University of Central England and Affiliated Consultant at the Institute of Reflective Practice, UK.

Sue Lillyman is a qualified nurse and midwife who worked in clinical practice for many years in a variety of hospitals within the West Midlands region prior to entering nurse education in 1989. Recently she worked as a volunteer with street boys and provided medical care in the shantytowns of Lima and remote villages on the Amazon in Peru. Sue is currently working at the University of Central England as Senior Lecturer where she is the route director for the Post-graduate Certificate in the Case Management of Patients with Long-term Conditions.

Sue has had an interest in reflective practice and the improvement of patient care through reflection for many years and been involved with portfolio development of staff, accreditation of prior learning and professional development.

Sue is on the international advisory board of the peer-reviewed journal, *Reflective Practice*. Her work with the Institute of Reflective Practice is in the area of helping others reach full potential within their workplace through reflection and the development of reflective workplace cultures.

Debbie Peniket MSc, RGN, RM, RHV
Assistant Director of Nursing and Therapies, South Birmingham PCT.

Debbie Peniket's career in the NHS now spans some 30 years. She has worked in general nursing, midwifery and health visiting and is currently an Assistant Director of Nursing and Therapies in South Birmingham PCT.

Most of her experience is within community services as a general health visitor and as a specialist health visitor for people with physical disabilities. This sparked her interest in the management of long-term neurological conditions and she undertook a Masters Degree in Advanced Clinical Practice at the University of Birmingham in 1998. Following this, Debbie worked as a nurse consultant until September 2003 when she took up her current post as an assistant director of nursing and therapies. She has a lead role in safeguarding Children and is a member of the Birmingham Safeguarding Children Board. In addition she is the trust lead for essence of care and the implementation of clinical supervision. Debbie provides facilitation for a leadership development programme and is involved in the modernisation of community services to deliver high quality, effective and patient/client-centred services.

Acknowledgements

Sue Lillyman and Tony Ghaye would like to thank all their colleagues and friends who have worked with them over the years in the implementation of clinical supervision and given their time and ideas in relation to this revised book.
They also thank Karen Latimer and Debbie Peniket for contributing chapters, and the staff and students within the trusts who have participated in action learning sets, clinical supervision sessions, staff surveys and steering groups to implement forms of clinical supervision, and who have shared its value in practice.

Introduction

Since the first edition of this book there have been developments in the process of clinical supervision with the onset of the health care standards set out by the Department of Health (2006). This document requires every NHS trust to meet these standards for their governance objectives in relation to leadership and clinical supervision. Although having some kind of process of clinical supervision in place in a trust is important, we see its real value as lying, not only in the objectives of the organisation, but also for the patient/client and individual practitioner. A fully functioning clinical supervision process clearly demonstrates a trust's commitment to improving the quality of its services by supporting all its staff. Such a process also sends a powerful message to service users. That there is a formal process in place where staff can explore new and better ways of providing the best quality of care for them.

In this book we have revisited the reasons why clinical supervision was first suggested as an important process and identified areas where we feel there has been a positive move towards its implementation. The book identifies how individuals and groups can positively engage in such a process and how this in turn contributes to their efforts to be life-long learners. We link clinical supervision with the knowledge and skills dimensions as set in the Department of Health's document (2004) and individual's development plans/portfolios.

In this edition we build on the first book and review where we are now in relation to the implementation of support networks for all professionals. We also identify why some parts of the process of clinical supervision have not lived up to their early promise and raise some new possibilities for both an appropriate conception of clinical supervision and its implementation.

Sue Lillyman
Tony Ghaye

Department of Health (2004) *The NHS Knowledge and Skills Framework and the Development Review Process*. London, HMSO
Department of Health (2006) *Standards for Better Health*. London, HMSO

CHAPTER I

What clinical supervision means to the practitioner, patient and organisation

Sue Lillyman

Introduction

This chapter reviews some of the reasons why clinical supervision was first introduced into the health care arena and its continued value for the individual practitioner, profession and organisation.

Clinical supervision can be used to develop individual practitioners' practice, and to help them achieve their plans and meet requirements for professional portfolios. Clinical supervision can enhance patient/client care through competent and safe practitioners, and organisations can benefit through improved health care standards and improved retention of staff.

The origins of clinical supervision

Many of us have heard and/or been part of clinical supervision over the past few decades but it is useful to identify where the process began. Rolf *et al* (2001) note its origins in the psychoanalytic work of Sigmund Freud in the 1920s. They also note the later work of Carl Rogers who expanded the idea and used it with counsellors and psychotherapists.

Its concept was introduced into the NHS through the Government's *Vision for the Future* (National Health Service Management Executive, 1993) which described it as:

> *A process of professional support and learning which enables individual practitioners to develop knowledge and competence, assume responsibility for their own practice and enhance consumer protection and safety of care in complex clinical situations.*
>
> (National Health Service Management Executive, 1993)

The United Kingdom Central Council for Nurses Midwives and Health Visitors, at the time, included it in their *Code of Professional Practice* (1992a) and the *Scope of Professional Practice* (1992b). Other professional groups have also taken the process on board to meet their own professional requirements and NHS trusts have included it in their strategies. The National Health Service Management Executive (1993) and the Kings Fund (1995) advocated clinical supervision as good practice.

The need for clinical supervision was highlighted again following several reports on poor practice, including the Beverley Allit inquiry (Clothier *et al*, 1994), the inquiry into Harold Shipman, and the Bristol Inquiry (Bristol Royal Infirmary Inquiry, 2001). Although we will never know if clinical supervision would have made a difference in the outcome of the events that led up to these inquiries, it may have provided the arena for staff to review their practice and perhaps given them the courage to speak up a little earlier. It would also have helped the practitioners through a difficult time following the events and provided support for those staff who had to deal with their feelings and media interest.

The role then developed with the Department of Health's (1999) *Making a Difference* document where it was stated that clinical supervision was integral to an organisational clinical governance strategy. This was reinforced in 2000 by the Department of Health in the *NHS Plan* (Department of Health, 2000). Finally, with the introduction of the health care standards (Department of Health, 2006) NHS trusts now have to identify where standards are being met in relation to clinical supervision.

Although the need for clinical supervision has been noted over the past few decades and it has been identified as good practice there are still only pockets of supervision being undertaken and they are not always linked to critical reflection or innovations in practice (Bond and Holland, 1998).

The changing names of clinical supervision

As the process has developed and moved into the wider health care setting its name has changed in many NHS trusts to incorporate more than clinical practitioners. The original name 'clinical supervision' suggested that it applied only to those working in a 'clinical' setting and 'supervision' implied some observation of care delivery. To get away from this perception and suggest a more supportive process many NHS trusts have used the term 'practice support'. This new title embraces all staff working within the NHS, including office workers, porters, gardeners and community staff as well as clinicians, and recognises that all staff work together for clients/ patients. It recognises that all staff working within the NHS require support and through that support are able to continue to develop and learn from their practice.

What is clinical supervision?

Voluntary

Although the pressure is on NHS trusts to identify where clinical supervision is being undertaken in order to achieve their health care standards, clinical supervision should be a voluntary process. If this process is not voluntary then it will not work, as practitioners may view it as a management process and consequently may not feel comfortable discussing issues that affect their practice.

Before commencing the process it is important that staff members know and understand the process and the value it will have for them as individuals as well as to patients and the organisation.

Non-prescriptive

The process is non-prescriptive in its approach. As we know different people have different learning styles and respond to different approaches. This is discussed further below where some models and how they can be used in different approaches to clinical supervision are reviewed.

Models of approach

There are several models of approach to clinical supervision including:

- *One-to-one*. This approach includes two people, a supervisor and supervisee. They meet together on a given date and at a specific time. The supervisor may be a peer or someone with experience in the field of practice that can guide and reflect on the issues raised by the supervisee.
- *Group*. Group supervision normally includes up to six staff members who meet together to share common issues across a team. A supervisor usually guides the process but this role may be rotated around the group to assist with role development and allow all team members to take part in the process. The group may consist of staff from a given area, ie. all from the same office, ward, health centre, etc., or from one speciality sharing common issues such as newly qualified staff, managers, etc. The group can be made up of people from the same discipline or may be multi-professional. The group can use a clinical supervision model/ process or work as an action learning set. The latter is discussed fully in *Chapter 5*.
- *Networking/peer*. The final model is that of networking with

practitioners outside the trust or across the trust. This model is appropriate where people work in isolation or in specialist areas. Group members may seek supervision with a similar practitioner outside their own workplace.

What clinical supervision is not

Managerial control

Supervision is not a managerial control system where a manager can enquire about practice or set an agenda for the meeting. It is a confidential meeting between supervisee(s) and supervisor to review practice, reflect on it and then either celebrate or change practice in light of the reflection and learning.

Hierarchical in nature

Ideally the sessions should not be hierarchical in nature where the supervisor is the person in authority. Supervisees should be encouraged to select their own supervisor and may choose a peer rather than someone in authority. In group supervision sessions, the role of supervisor may rotate around a group of peers. The supervisor is there to guide the process not to dictate the contents of the session.

Appraisal

It is not an appraisal or an individual process review; neither does clinical supervision take the place of these. However, supervisees may use the reflections to achieve their goals set at their individual process review/appraisal.

Another hurdle to get over

The main issue in relation to the failure of clinical supervision to date has been the lack of understanding and time commitment that people feel they are able to give to the process. To some this appears to be yet another hurdle they have to cross in their busy schedules and therefore they are not committed to the process. However, if developed and used correctly clinical supervision can assist practitioners to achieve other aspects of their development including development plans for their knowledge and skills framework (Department of Health, 2004) and continual professional development portfolios required for professional bodies, for example the post-registration education and practice requirements for nurses and midwives (Nursing and Midwifery Council, 2004). This is discussed later in this chapter.

Counselling

Supervisors may find themselves using counselling skills in the session. However, supervisors must be aware that supervisees need to be referred to a counselling service should issues arise outside the supervisor's ability.

Confessional

The process is not for people to confess or blow the whistle on colleagues. There are other processes within the trust should people feel they wish to do this. Neither is the process just to review where supervisees feel their practice is not up to standard. Indeed there is an element here where good practice can be celebrated through the reflective process.

The process of clinical supervision

Bishop and Freshwater (2000) and Clouder and Sellars (2004) note differences of opinion about the rationale, and uncertainties about how the process should be operationalised. Hasebo and Kihlgren (2004) agree that there is no single method/process of implementation. However, most authors agree that it is a means to improve a person's competence and skills (Matthews and Altman, 1997; Rundqvist and Severinsson, 1999).

People must enter the process as volunteers. It was Lewin in 1963 who claimed that people who make their own decisions are more motivated than people who are the passive targets of forces imposed from outside. Adequate training for the role of both supervisor and supervisee needs to be undertaken so that participants understand the roles and their value to both the individual and organisation. Training should include the supervisors' need to be able to consider the principles on which they work rather than working on their skills (Fish and Twin, 1997).

It is a formal agreement where two or more practitioners (depending on the chosen model) meet to discuss their work on a regular basis. The meeting usually takes place four to six weekly and takes one to two hours depending on the group and availability of staff. It involves reflecting on practice in order to learn from that practice to improve competency (Kings Fund, 1995).

The purpose of clinical supervision

As stated by Fish and Twin (1997), practice is not a simple task or skill. It is a complex, dynamic and social activity that is underpinned by sets of values and beliefs, and traditions and theoretical perceptions that include moral dimensions. Clinical supervision can help practitioners as they attempt to deal with all these aspects in their everyday life. Through this process of practitioners supporting each other the main purpose has ultimately to be to improve the quality of patient care (Butterworth and Woods, 1998). If participants reflect critically on their practice and develop action plans, they are arguably better able to deliver informed knowledge-based practice (Johns, 2004). They are able to understand the origins of practice and unravel some of the complexities and underlying theoretical concepts. They may be able to articulate and understand why they do things in a certain way and identify areas where they are constrained due to certain organisational policies, values and beliefs.

Safeguarding standards of care, as identified in the Allit, Shipman and Bristol reports, requires clinical supervision and support for staff. In the reports of these inquries it was suggested that staff be provided with a safe environment where they can raise issues of concern and discuss confidential issues that might in return lead to poor practice being identified sooner.

Clinical supervision also assists practitioners with their development of professional expertise. Benner (1984) used the novice-to-expert range of practice. She suggested that at registration practitioners are competent in the skills and knowledge to carry out a role. However, once a person is qualified there is a requirement to develop that practice to an expert level of delivery. Although academic study may fill some of the gaps in knowledge and theoretical aspects of practice, professional development comes from practice itself. It is through critical reflection on practice that professionals can then move their practice forward, develop new skills and identify the gaps in their knowledge base. Sometimes we do not always know what we do not know and through reflection we can identify where that knowledge is lacking, especially if we have an informed supervisor who can assist in unravelling the complexities of practice.

Some benefits

For the practitioner

Most professionals want to do their job to the best of their ability and to develop to an expert level in their chosen field. Through clinical supervision, as stated above, practitioners can develop their roles and identify where there are gaps in their own professional development, identify where they require further formal education or seek their own answers to practice. It can assist practitioners in their continuing professional development and help them gain evidence for their professional portfolio and knowledge and skills framework development plan through written reflections following supervision sessions.

Supervision has also been reported as a protection and advocacy process that is linked with change and conflict for the practitioner (Kirkham and Stapleton, 2000).

For the patient/client

If patients feel practitioners understand their roles and are competent they will benefit from their expertise and feel confident and gain trust in them (Butterworth and Woods, 1998).

For the organisation

The organisation is likely to see improved quality of patient care with reduced complaints and hopefully a reduction in bad practice. Members of staff are less likely to go off sick or leave the profession if they feel supported and have been given time for their own needs (Butterworth *et al*, 1996; Berg and Halberg, 1999). Finally the organisation will be able to identify where it can achieve its governance targets and heath care standards.

Is clinical supervision working?

Clinical supervision is well established in social work and mental health nursing through caseload work in line with the Mental Health Act of 1993. Midwifery has also had supervision since 1936 when the role of inspector changed to supervisor. However, this has been linked to a managerial process. Midwifery is now reviewing this role as supervision as support. Psychology and counselling professionals also undertake weekly supervision sessions as a prerequisite of their code of ethics (British Association for Counselling, 1993).

In nursing and allied health care professions clinical supervision is not well established and many feel it is not working due to the confusion surrounding the process, fear of disempowerment and critical intrusion of their practice (Bond and Holland, 1998).

Also there has been a failure on the part of organisations who may not provide protected time for staff to meet for clinical supervision, especially where they do not see the value for the organisation.

In a recent survey (Lillyman, 2006) it was encouraging to note that 47% ($n = 217$) of practitioners had undergone training for clinical supervision, 62% were currently engaged in clinical supervision and 65% included networking, action-learning sets, peer support and professional groups as part of their support networks. Although the support process is not always seen as clinical supervision there are other methods of support being undertaken by staff as noted in their responses. In order to fulfil the requirements of continual development of the practitioner and the governance agenda for the organisation these other support processes need to be identified and recognised.

Some models of supervision and support

Growth and support model

Faugier (1992) developed the growth and support model where the supervisor facilitates growth both educationally and personally in the supervisee. Supervisors provide essential support to their supervisees' developing clinical autonomy. The supervisor is therefore responsible for the following elements of the relationship:

- generosity
- rewarding
- openness
- willingness to learn
- thoughtfulness and thought provoking
- humanity
- sensitivity
- personal
- practical
- orientation
- relationship
- trust.

Integrative approach

An integrative approach was suggested by Hawkins and Shohet (1989). This approach looks more closely at the process of the supervisory relationship and divides supervision into four main components

- supervisor
- client
- supervisee
- work context.

They interlock the process into two systems: the therapy system that connects the client and supervisee and the supervision system that involves the supervisee and supervisor. Both systems are based on similar types of an agreed contract of time spent together with negotiated shared tasks and goals.

Interactive model

Proctor (1992) developed what she referred to as a three function interactive model. The three components consisted of:

- *Normative* (managerial) where there is promotion of and complying with policies and procedures, developing standards and contributing to clinical audit.
- *Formative* (educative) where skills are developed and evidence based on nursing practice.
- *Restorative* (pastoral support) enabling practitioners to understand and manage the emotional stress of practice.

She suggests that all the elements of these three components must be considered integral parts of an evaluation system for the process of clinical supervision.

Other models noted by Rolfe *et al* (2001) include:

Psychodynamic model

The psychodynamic model is taken from the work of Sigmund Freud where human behaviour is governed by unconscious factors. This involves a therapeutic relationship and may include the transference of feelings about a client to the supervisor. The supervisor needs to be aware that feelings being displayed towards them such as anger may be the way a supervisee is feeling towards other people and should not take this personally. This model however does offer strict boundaries and clear contract setting for the participants. The role is on self and knowing self in relation to others and results in a potential shift in self-image. As suggested earlier this is where the blind window of the Johari window (see p. 13) might start to be exposed.

Humanistic model

The humanistic model is rooted in the work of Carl Rogers (1969) and is more person centred in its approach. The core conditions of empathy, genuineness and respect or unconditional regard are necessary for effective individual respect. Building a relationship based on trust between the participants leads to more autonomous and responsible practitioners. The supervisor empowers supervisees to take their practice forward with a non-judgemental approach. This approach is seen in the action learning sets discussed in *Chapter 5*.

Systemic model

The systemic model is based on the idea that there are many possible ways of looking at reality and that there is no ultimate objective truth. The session is influenced by the context and social background of the individual, patient and organisation. The supervision set explores all the possibilities without concluding one process or practice as the answer.

Roles of the supervisor

Once the process has been agreed by the organisation and time given for staff to attend some form of supervision, the staff members need some training in relation to the process, its value and the role they will play. The supervisor and supervisee will require different training programmes if the organisation sees their roles as different.

The supervisor is responsible for the practical aspects of the session such as programming the meeting on a four to six weekly basis and helping the group to set its own ground rules in relation to confidentiality, responsibility, commitment, respect and time keeping. The supervisor will also take on the role of time keeping and the supervision process, helping practitioners to reflect critically on their practice and develop an action plan for future development.

Supervisors also need to be aware of the model adopted, as discussed above, and their own approach in relation to the way they supervise the session. As Heron (1975) noted there are different approaches, such as the supervisor who is authoritative or directive, or prescriptive, informative and confrontational as against supervisors who are cathartic, catalytic and supportive. Supervisors need to use their skills but be concerned for the supervisees while using authority to ensure goals are met.

The supervisor also needs to be aware of the communication strategies that can be used by people and/or groups and therefore we will explore some known strategies that people might use within groups. The supervisor needs to be aware of what is going on and guide the group in a constructive and meaningful meeting.

Communication models

When supervising a session there are several models that the supervisor needs to be aware of. Two models are presented here: Berne's (1966) transactional analysis and the Johari window (Luft, 1969).

Transactional analysis

Berne (1966) postulated that we interact using three different ego states, that of adult, child and parent, based on our behaviour in relation to an immediate experience. These states are nothing to do with our age or position. All three states are used depending on where people are and with whom they are communicating. We can use the state to manipulate situations, change other people's perceptions and play games with each other. It is therefore important that supervisors recognise where supervisees are coming from and if games are being played within the meeting. They can then guide the session to include appropriate levels of communication. Also supervisors need to be aware of their own ego state as this too could affect the interaction and learning that is going on in the session. Different ego states can create a good environment in which we can learn or they can destroy it.

Berne suggested we could present at different times in the parent, child and adult ego state.

The parent

This state is made up of two aspects: the critical/controlling and nurturing parent. The parent state is the source of our values, judgements, prohibitions and our normative world with a clear sense of responsibility.

The critical parent is as it suggests, where people use their communication in such a way as to take charge of the situation and in doing so may have strong opinions and may be prejudiced and judgemental. The critical parent is not open to other people's opinions. This may lead to supervisees becoming less confident in their practice and undervaluing themselves. On the other hand the nurturing parent supports and is protective and sympathetic. This might result in not allowing supervisees to develop and grow on their own. Nurturing parents may provide what they feel is required, putting over their own interpretation of events and not allowing supervisees to develop and reflect on their own situation and draw their own conclusions.

The child

This ego state, Berne suggests, is dominated by emotions and feelings commonly associated with childhood. It is divided into three sub-ego states and includes the adoptive, little professor and free child. The adopted child wants to please and therefore will react in the way he or she thinks the other person wants them to act. This might be in response to the nurturing parent. Again learning situations may be lost if the person in the child state is trying to please the supervisor and not getting down to the real issues that might be affecting their work.

The little professor is the inquisitive and creative child who is always looking for answers, taking things to pieces and trying to rebuild. Supervisees in this ego state need direction as they might go off in all directions and fail to get to the bottom of an issue before they begin working on something else. Free children are impulsive and display anger if they do not get their own way; they are often not open to guidance in their reflections or practice.

The adult

Characterised by rational thought, information processing and the facility of checking and comparing with past experience, this is the ego state that supervisors should be guiding their supervisees and themselves into. This state reflects the person who respects others and searches in partnership with others for answers. If this state can reached for both parties then real exploration of solutions and answers can be achieved. There will be a partnership in the relationship and both will feel comfortable with the process.

Berne then identifies four life positions:

I am not ok – you are ok
In this situation people tend to accept a psychologically inferior position in relation to others. There is a lack of confidence and self-worth in this position if the supervisee who looks up to the supervisor takes on this position.

I am not ok – you are not ok
In this situation people believe they are worthless and also view everyone else the same. If this occurs in the supervisor it can lead to an alienation from others including the supervisee with little sense of purpose in the process or the communication.

I am ok – you are not ok
Here people feel they cannot rely on anyone else and want to do things on their own. They often perceive the situation they are in as someone else's fault with little insight into their own behaviour.

I am ok – you are ok
This life position is where there is a competent and interdependent relationship with others. People are competent in their own ability, respect others and work in partnership with others. Here the reflective process can progress and issues can be addressed by all involved in the supervision session.

Johari window

Luft (1969) developed the Johari window for communication and note that each person has four parts or windows. This is a useful model for the supervisor who can identify where supervisees are coming from and help them to discover areas unknown to themselves.

The Johari window consists of the open window, the hidden self, the blind and the unknown. The open self is that part of us that we share with others; we are willing for others to know certain aspects of our lives and will discuss these freely in the clinical supervision session. The supervisor needs to recognise that this area is shared willingly; it may be quite small when starting the group and as people gain the trust and respect of others it will open up more.

The hidden self is where people keep certain aspects of their life to themselves. Again as the group develops there is often more disclosure and this area will be opened up further when deeper and honest reflections can be engaged. The supervisor must be aware of when and how much people are opening themselves up as they may become vulnerable. If the situation is not handled well it may result in people closing the window.

The unknown self is where people might have little insight into their own behaviour and not recognise what is happening as a result of it. Here the supervisor needs to open up that self without hurting or embarrassing people but allowing them to gain insight into their own behaviour. This can be achieved through feedback to the person. This might be evident when discussing a situation where personalities are clashing and the people presenting fail to see their own input into the situation but others may feel that they understand why things are happening.

The last window is the closed window of which people themselves are unaware as are others around them. During the sessions some aspects may open up to both parties as deeper reflection is engaged.

Supervisors must never push supervisees beyond their safe boundaries but encourage them to open up some aspects that can then be developed. Although there is some danger in this approach it is for supervisors to be sensitive to what is going on with their supervisees and support them through any issues that may arise.

To make more sense of the situation and find out more about ourselves we need to make use of and relate effectively to other people.

The role of the supervisee

As we can see the role of the supervisee is not subservient but rather a partnership where supervisees work together with their supervisor to reflect critically on an issue or aspect of practice and identify an action plan or learning that can be derived from that situation. As already stated supervision is voluntary and supervisees should be able to choose their supervisor as someone they feel confident with. They should have trust in their ability to support them through their practice. Supervisees should be open to the process and have a willingness to learn from their practice. They need to develop critical reflection with their supervisor and be honest in the process. There is an equal responsibility for the supervisor and supervisee in monitoring, evaluating and setting the agenda for the session.

Clinical governance and clinical supervision

NHS trusts have to demonstrate their provision of and staff involvement in clinical supervision in order to achieve their health care standards (Department of Health, 2006). For this reason staff may be required to maintain records of the time spent and names of the people involved in a session. The contents of the session, as stated, are confidential to the people taking part and should not be requested by the trust. Each trust will be required to complete an audit of staff being supervised in order to achieve health care standards and are requested to complete action plans to achieve and monitor them.

Knowledge and skills framework and continuing professional development plans

As stated earlier clinical supervision is not just another time-consuming process to add to a busy schedule but can, if used correctly, support the knowledge and skills framework and requirements for continuing professional development.

During clinical supervision supervisees can make notes of their practice and how they have reflected and developed through the session. Using these reflective writings they can provide evidence for both professional development profiles and the knowledge and skills framework requirements if they take into account the dimensions they need to achieve. All these assist practitioners to become proficient in their role and together can provide the evidence to support those claims.

A way forward

As NHS trusts produce their individual strategies they need to include staff development along with quality provision and the improvement of patient care. Job descriptions and audits also need to include the provision of clinical supervision. Training for staff to act as supervisors and supervisees needs to be in place to identify the processes stated in this chapter before supervision can fulfil the requirements for the individual, profession and organisation.

References

Benner P (1984) *From Novice to Expert*. Addison-Wesley, Menlo Park

Berg A, Halberg IR (1999) Effects of systematic clinical supervision on psychiatric nurse' sense of coherence, creativity, work related strain, job satisfaction and view of the effects from clinical supervision: A pre-post test design. *Journal of Psychiatric and Mental Health Nursing*: 371–81

Berne E (1966) *Games People Play*. Andre Deutsch, London

Bishop V, Freshwater D (2000) *Clinical Supervision: Examples and Pointers for Good Practice*. Unpublished report for University Leicester Hospitals Education.

Bristol Royal Infirmary Inquiry (2001) *Final report: Learning from Bristol: The Report of the Public Inquiry into Children's Heart Surgery at Bristol Royal Infirmary 1984–1995*. Command Paper CM 5207 BRI Inquiry Bristol

Bond M, Holland S (1998) *Skills of Clinical Supervision for Nurses*. Open University Press, Milton Keynes

British Association for Counselling (1993) *The Code of Ethics and Practice for Counsellors*. British Association for Counselling, London

Butterworth T, Woods D (1998) *Clinical Governance and Clinical Supervision: Working Together to Ensure Safe and Accountable Practice – a Briefing Paper*. Manchester, University of Manchester

Butterworth T, Bishop V, Carson J (1996) First steps towards evaluating clinical supervision in nursing and health visiting: Theory, policy and practice development. A review. *J Clin Nurs* **5**: 127–32

Clothier C, MacDonald C, Shaw D (1994) *Independent Inquiry into Deaths and Injuries on the Children's Ward at Grantham and Kesteven General Hospital During the Period February to April 1991* (Allitt Inquiry). London, HMSO

Clouder L, Sellars J (2004) Reflective practice and clinical supervision: An interprofessional perspective. *J Adv Nurs* **46**(3): 262–9

Department of Health (1999) *Making a Difference*. London, HMSO

Department of Health (2000) *Meeting the Challenge. A Strategy for Allied Health Professionals*. London, HMSO

Department of Health (2004) *The NHS Knowledge and Skills Framework and the development review process*. London, HMSO

Department of Health (2006) *Standards for Better Health*. London, HMSO

Faugier J (1992) The supervisory relationship in clinical supervision and mentorship in nursing. In Butterworth T, Faugier J (eds) *Clinical Supervision and Mentorship in Nursing*. London, Chapman and Hall

Fish D, Twin S (1997) *Quality Clinical Supervision in the Health Care Professions*. Oxford, Butterworth Heinemann

Hasebo G, Kihlgren M (2004) Nursing Home Care: Changes after Supervision *J Adv Nurs* **45**(3): 269–79

Hawkins P, Shohet, R (1989) *Supervision in the Helping Professions*. Milton Keynes, Open University Press

Heron J (1975) *Six Category Interventions Analysis*. Guildford, University of Surrey

Kirkham M, Stapleton H (2000) Midwives' support needs as childbirth changes. *J Adv Nurs* **32**(2): 465–72

King's Fund (1995) *Clinical Supervision: An Executive summary*. London, King's Fund

Johns C (2004) *Becoming a Reflective Practitioner* (2nd edn). Oxford, Blackwell Publishing

Lewin K (1963) *Field Theory in Social Science: Selected Theoretical Papers*. London, Tavistock

Lillyman S (2006) *Practice Support (Clinical Supervision) Survey of staff Report January 2006*. Unpublished report. Birmingham, SBPCT

Luft J (1969) *Of Human Interaction*. Palo Alto, The National Press

Nursing and Midwifery Council (2004) *The PREP Handbook*. London, Nursing and

Midwifery Council

Matthews RM, Altman H (1997) Teaching nurse aids to promote independence in people with dementia. *J Clin Geropsychol* **3**: 149–59

NHS Management Executive (1993) *A Vision for the Future*. London, HMSO.

Proctor B (1992) *Supervision in the Helping Professions*. Milton Keynes, Open University Press.

Rolfe G, Freshwater D, Jasper M (2001) *Critical Reflection for Nursing and the Helping Professions: A Users Guide*. Hampshire, Palgrove Macmillan.

Rogers C (1969) *Freedom to Learn*. Ohio, Merrill

Rundgvist EM, Severinsson EI (1999) Caring relationships with patients suffering from dementia – An interview study. *J Adv Nurs* **29**: 800–7

United Kingdom Central Council for Nursing, Midwifery and Health Visiting (1992a) *Code of Professional Conduct for the Nurse, Midwife and Health Visitor*. London, UKCC

United Kingdom Central Council for Nursing, Midwifery and Health Visiting (1992b) *The Scope of Professional Practice*. London, UKCC

CHAPTER 2

Clinical supervision: ethics and appreciative interaction

Tony Ghaye

An NHS trust in the UK was recently reflecting upon its Dignity at Work Policy. The reason for this was an increasing number of complaints, allegedly, about bullying. Apparently these were being dealt with through the trust's informal and formal procedures. The trust also had a process of one-to-one clinical supervision in place. Conversations about bullying were also being presented through this process. Twice a year all the supervisors came together for a 'learning day'. During one such event, one supervisor said the following. What feelings and thoughts does it trigger in your mind?

I've had a number of colleagues come to me to talk about bullying at work, about being bullied themselves and about witnessing bullying. So our clinical supervision sessions have been about this. One colleague who said that she'd been bullied herself, talked about the need for more attention to be paid to staff who are experiencing problems like this. She said that persistent bullies are only getting told off. Another talked about her wish for all kinds of intimidation and bullying to be stamped out. She said that she had experienced being bullied by a senior staff member in the organisation. She used the word victimisation.

The worst conversation I've had was when a colleague came to me and said, 'We just have to stop the incessant back-stabbing, bitching and blaming culture that is absolutely rife in this department. New (and old) staff are treated by some senior staff like dirt, and we have already lost some fantastic staff to bullying and (apparently) respect-demanding egomaniacs. I've been bullied so I know how others feel. It's terrible. Awful. It makes me so upset. I've had people speak in such a patronising way, spiteful really. Why do they have to be like this? I've had my confidence really knocked back. Why did she have to say, "I'm surprised you couldn't do that", …and in that way, and in front of my patient? She always has a go. She picks on me. Why me? I'm so glad I've got a loving husband. He restores my faith in me because I'm certainly not valued at work.

Well that's how it feels. How can we give the best care we can when we don't feel valued and respected?'

This supervisor was describing some very uncomfortable experiences. Uncomfortable not only for those coming to the supervisor and using their clinical supervision sessions to air such feelings but also for the supervisor. So what issues are raised here and what lessons can be learnt from them?

One central issue is an ethical one. How far can we claim that our practices of clinical supervision are ethical? Why does it matter that we are ethical? What does it mean to be ethical, unethical and who says so? One answer is because being ethical is about how we treat our fellow human beings and, in the context of clinical supervision, how we best meet our colleagues' learning needs. There are many things going on in this supervisor's statement. It is full of ethical dilemmas, for example about rights to autonomy, confidentiality, anonymity, dignity, respectfulness, being valued, professional competence, inter-personal conflicts, fairness, conflicting loyalties, discipline, and encroachments on personal liberty. And what about, 'only do unto others what you would like them to do to you'? For many people, this is the only ethical principal they know, even if they do not describe it in this way.

A second central issue is an appreciative one. If you take the process of clinical supervision to be about the conscious co-creation of meaning, then it follows that the dynamics of our relationship with our supervisor (or in the context of group supervision, with our peers) is crucial. If 'problems' such as those described above are being presented during such sessions, there is a real danger that the conversation between participants becomes deficit-based. By this I mean we spend a lot of time and energy talking about and trying to work out ways to get rid of the 'problem'. We try to 'fix' things. I am not saying that we should not use clinical supervision to discuss problems. What I am saying is that if the conversations are only about problems, we may be missing a real opportunity to try to see the best in one another and create new and better clinical practice together. So in this chapter I want to respond to the question, 'How can we do clinical supervision ethically and appreciatively?' I will suggest that it is important for us to understand the supervision process as one of applied ethics and appreciative interaction.

Applied ethics

The sentimental supervisor

Hollway (1991) argues that we are culturally coded as over-emotional. We are sentimental workers. Given this, it is perhaps surprising to note that there are still relatively few accounts of supervision processes that clearly link feeling, thinking and action. There may be many reasons for this. I will cluster some together. One may be the (still) pervasive notion that clinical supervision is essentially a cognitive activity. Another may be the enduring Deweyian (after John Dewey) belief that supervision is essentially a problem-solving process that begins with something that is perplexing, disturbing or worrying. Another might be the view that, 'cognition and rationality are usually seen as outside of, or superior to, emotions' (Swan and Bailey, 2004: 106). Another might be associated with the positivist predilection for separating reason from emotion and values and subjectivities from situated action. This kind of thinking is based upon dichotomy and binary opposition. We see it everywhere in Western societies. 'We talk about right and wrong, nature and nurture, public or private, heart or head, quality or quantity; and of course, rational or emotional' (Carr, 2001: 421). When we use language like this, we elevate one term while simultaneously inferring a denigration of the other.

Emotionality in the process of clinical supervision

Clinical supervision is an example of reflective practice or, more specifically and frequently, reflection on practice (Schön, 1983). What comes with this belief is a view that we should not underestimate the emotionality involved in the process of conducting supervision. In other words, the nature, intensity and role in learning that emotion plays. For example, a common kind of practice, which Schön (1983) called reflection on action, requires us to re-experience something of past significance. Something significant might be a wonderful experience or something much less positive (eg. being bullied at work). In both cases, and with everything in between, there is an emotional content. Raelin (2001) suggests that emotions can act as catalysts for reflection. If we feel an aspect of our work, or a particular workplace encounter, made us feel jubilant and up-lifted, we might reflect on the reasons why we felt that way, if only to try to create conditions, or develop behaviours that enable us to feel this way again. The clinical supervision process can also generate emotions. If we reflect on an aspect of our work, a painful truth might emerge about it. May be there is a sense of powerlessness (Parry, 2003) or a feeling that we are not coping well with the pressures of work. Brookfield (1994) talks in some detail about the way certain kinds of reflective practice can generate feelings of anxiety, insecurity, sadness and loss. So I am suggesting that clinical supervision must come with a health warning.

Emotional 'display'

How can we develop an ethical interest in emotion and clinical supervision? They are inter-related, interactive and interdependent. Through the process of supervision we may find ourselves at the interface between emotion and learning, between feelings and ideas, between right and wrong and even having to confront two rights.. We need to be clear about which conception of emotion we are using. De Rivera (1977) offers three views.

- *Emotion as a psychological state*: For example a sense of well-being or frustration.
- *Emotion as a perception of value*: For example a feeling of gratitude to someone for being kind, or a feeling of anger in response to someone being inconsiderate towards us or demanding something that we are unable to give.
- *Emotion as transformation*: For example an experience or encounter at work that enhances self or collective understanding and helps us to improve what we are doing for our clients and patients.

In the example of bullying at work, it seems emotion is being placed firmly in a social and organisational context. Additionally the supervisor seems to be articulating a value position of clinical supervision being used as a 'site' of emotional 'display' as part of an intra and inter-personal, meaning-creating process.

Emotions can be pleasant and exciting (positive) or unpleasant and disturbing (negative). The social, institutional and cultural contexts we find ourselves in provide the rules and vocabularies of emotional 'display' for different audiences: self, loved one, boss, supervisor and so on (Antonacopoulou and Gabriel, 2001). So what rules and vocabularies should we discuss and use in order to maximise the learning opportunities between supervisor and supervisee? Are there, for example, some feelings that we cannot express to our personal satisfaction? Is it possible that supervisees might be able to express feelings which others (eg. their supervisors) find difficult to understand? What would be the process for both to have an appreciative conversation (Ghaye, 2007) about the constructive alignment (or contradictions) between feelings, thinking and actions? In emotionally loaded supervision sessions, we should be careful not to muddy the water between feelings that are willed and judged and those suffered, coped with and submitted to. I am touching the tips of at least two large icebergs here. One might be called pathos, the other logos. Antonacopoulou and Gabriel (2001: 441–2) said,

Adults cannot be considered emotionally developed unless they understand the significance of emotion in representing their self-feelings, anticipate the effects of these feelings in a social context and identify and respond to the feelings of others.'

In the process of supervision we often make assumptions about the emotional competence (Kolb *et al*, 1986) of those who are engaging in it. If a purpose of clinical supervision is to enhance learning, we need to understand fully the interdependence of learning and emotion. Learning may contain, reframe and transform emotion; but it is itself shaped by emotion.

Five ethical capacities to display through clinical supervision

Einhorn (2006) suggests that we have five capacities (he calls them tools) which enable us to be ethical. They are:

- Using already developed norms, rules and laws and using them as guiding lights. In this case it might be participant understanding of the 'rules' governing the trust's supervision process, for example regarding the what, where, how often and with whom aspects. Also it might be about its documentation and possible impact on the individual, clinical team or organisation.
- Using our ability to reason and so act rationally. This involves evaluating which actions will do as much good as possible and how to avoid doing harm. I suggest there is a joint responsibility, when engaging in the supervision process, for all concerned to reflect before acting (or speaking).
- Using our conscience which can act as an inner compass and an emotional indicator about what might make us feel good or bad.
- Using our capacity to empathise and in so doing, put ourselves in someone else's place.
- Using our relationships with others as a source of advice, as sounding boards and as a source of comfort. This also means that we need to pay attention to where we place our attention and what we attend to in our supervisory conversation. It means being aware of how our attention is being shaped by and through others, and vice versa.

Clinical supervision as emotional labour

How far is successful supervision linked with our ability to engage emotionally and detach ourselves from the process, a process that is often emotionally loaded? If supervision is a caring process, it must involve feeling. A caring process may be emotionally demanding and personally challenging. In Hochschild's (1983) original description of the emotional labour of flight attendants, there is reference to the management of feeling and its public display, the 'putting on of a brave face'. This display might, for example be through facial expression of certain emotions as part of one's job. This is particularly prevalent in human service work. What would be the implications of regarding the clinical supervision process as an example of emotional labour? It is possible that a supervisee wants to 'disclose her personal feelings'. It is also possible that her supervisor has learnt how to switch on and off, to draw the line, to keep a bit of a barrier up, to keep some distance and perspective on things. In situations like this, how do we sustain the process as an ethical one? I suggest we need to think through the practicalities embraced within the dualism of engagement and detachment. We also need to be more explicit about the fundamental issue of the nature of our knowing.

Appreciative interaction

Using a language of positive regard through clinical supervision

The key attributes of a language of positive regard include the following. First, it is a language where the supervisee informs other participants of the significance of what it is they are bringing to the session, for them. Second, it is specific information about their personal experiences. Third, it is non-attributive, ie. the conversation focuses on the experience and not on particular members of staff that might have been involved in that experience. Fourth, it is potentially transformational for both the supervisee and for other participants, through the act of telling and listening. Finally, such conversations give all those involved the opportunity to communicate appreciation. So we need to ask, 'What processes are in place for a clinical supervision conversation of positive regard to happen?' This is not only about ethical aspects (as defined earlier) and their application. It is also about building and sustaining appreciative interactions.

Building a language of positive regard through trust

I have argued elsewhere (Ghaye, 2005) of the importance of trust for meaningful relationships and for improving services. Although it is complex to establish and sustain trust, it is usually assumed to be a prerequisite for most clinical supervision processes where building shared values, meanings and positive action is so important. Without trust, conversations of positive regard are non-starters. Reina and Reina (2006) help us understand the importance of trust (and betrayal) in the workplace and how this forms and transforms relationships. At the heart of their book is the notion of transactional trust. This is a process of mutual exchange, reciprocity and something created incrementally over time. In other words we have to trust in order to increase the likelihood that we will be trusted. Reina and Reina (2006) set out three types of transactional trust.

- *Contractual trust*: This is essentially a trust of character. It is people actually doing what they say they will do. It is about keeping agreements, honouring intentions and behaving consistently. These are issues for all involved in the supervision process.
- *Communication trust*: This is essentially a trust of disclosure. It is about people's willingness to share information, to tell the truth, admit mistakes, celebrate achievements and successes, maintain confidentiality, and give and receive constructive feedback. Trust influences the quality of our conversations and vice versa. It helps to build effective relationships with those with whom we work and who we care for. It connects us with one another and especially through a supervision process.
- *Competence trust*: This is essentially a trust of capability. How far do you trust the people you interact with during your supervision sessions? Do you trust them to give you an honest opinion about what it is you are bringing to the session? How capable do you feel they are in giving you constructive feedback? How capable are they in providing you with what you think you want and need to know in order to continue to better understand and maybe to improve your practice?

Building a language of positive regard through open listening

Kahane (2004) gives us a sharp reminder of the ways some interactions within health care organisations can go. He says, '

> The root of not listening is knowing. If I already know the truth, why do I need to listen to you? Perhaps out of politeness or guile I should pretend to listen, but what I really need to do is to tell you what I know, and if you don't listen, to tell you again, more forcefully. All authoritarian systems rest on the assumption that the boss can and does know the one right answer.
>
> (Kahane, 2004: 47).

Communication trust means talking openly and honestly. It brings with it a willingness and ability, on our part, to disclose to others, what is in our head and heart. Listening openly, on the other hand, means being willing and able to positively embrace something different and new from others. This is not as easy as it may sound because it involves issues about interpersonal relations, power, value alignment and so on. Listening sounds so simple. So I ask, 'When was the last time you felt you were listened to, openly, in a clinical supervision session? How do you know this? What made you feel this way? What were the circumstances that led up to this? What was the root cause of such a positive experience?'

Wheatley (2002) offers us some useful thoughts in what she eloquently describes as 'seeing how wise we can be together'. What we can learn from her work is that, to build supervision around conversations of positive regard, we not only have to learn to listen openly, but also to listen reflectively. Some of her thoughts are:

- *We need to learn how to acknowledge one another as equals*: A language of positive regard requires us to acknowledge that we are equal as human beings (unequal when in role) and that we need each other. We cannot always improve our practice or our clinical services by trying to figure things out on our own. This of course is an argument for group supervision.

- *We need to try to stay curious about each other*: We need to be genuinely interested in what we have to say to each other and not fearful. We need to test out our commitment to a value, 'I believe that I can learn something significant from you, each time I listen to you.' This weaves openness together with reflection.

- *We need to help each other to listen openly and then act appropriately*: It can be hard work to listen especially when we are busy and, even in a supervision session, we may find that our mind is wandering. It is hard to listen when we feel certain about something, or stressed. Try to think of a positive experience with your colleagues, when you know you listened to their views and then acted appropriately on them. What made this a positive experience?

- *We need to slow down to make time to listen reflectively*: If listening is an important part in developing a language of positive regard, so too is slowing down. Often we need to make time to listen to others' views in a supervision session and to reflect on them. Clinical supervision is not a business meeting with a crowded agenda.

- *We must expect it to be messy at times*: Conversations do not always move in a straight line. When learning from others through supervision, it is probable that some things do not appear to connect with our experiences and perceptions. Experiences can be diverse. Listening openly and reflectively means that we resist the impulse to tidy things up and put experiences in little boxes. We need to learn the benefits of being 'disturbed' and by this I mean having our ideas and practices challenged by others. How can we be creative in improving our practice and health care services if we are not willing to be disturbed? According to Kahane (2004: 83),

> To create new realities we have to listen reflectively. It is not enough to be able to hear clearly the chorus of other voices; we must also hear the contribution of our own voice. It is not enough to be able to see others

in the picture of what is going on; we must also see what we ourselves
are doing. It is not enough to be observers of the problem situation; we
must also recognise ourselves as actors who influence the outcome.'

Using the power of the positive question in clinical supervision

How can we shift the balance of conversations in supervisory sessions which
might be stuck with vocabularies around 'problems' and human deficit, and in so
doing, unlock the creative potential of staff who are participating in the process?
I ask this because we know that deficit-based questions (eg. 'How can we fix this
problem?') lead to deficit-based conversations, which in turn lead to deficit-based
patterns of action (Cooperrider and Whitney, 2005; Anderson *et al*, 2006). To
address this constructively we need to ask different kinds of questions to generate
different kinds of conversations in the supervision process.

Advocates of appreciative inquiry (Srivastva and Cooperrider, 1990;
Cooperrider and Whitney, 1999, 2003; Whitney and Trosten-Bloom, 2002;
Whitney *et al*, 2002; Cherney *et al*, 2004; Cooperrider *et al*, 2005) talk a lot
about the power of the positive question. Positive questions guide agendas
and focus attention in the direction of the aspects of organisational existence
– latent or explicit, historic or contemporary – that are most life-giving and life-
sustaining for employees. They are the kind of question that enable the creation
of powerful vocabularies of possibility, both in the day-to-day conversations of
staff and in the social and organisational theory that is produced about clinical
competence, service improvement and workplace transformation.

In this part of the chapter, I am stressing the centrality of the positive
question in clinical supervision and how it helps us avoid sessions becoming
preoccupied with deficits and problem-fixing actions. Gergen (1994) raises five
consequences of deficit-type conversations. I have interpreted them thus:

- *The containment of conversation*: Deficit-based conversations, as I have
  described them, often operate to establish a dualistic conversational
  structure in which this is opposed to that. For example, let us assume the
  argument is that flatter forms of organisational structure, or that sending
  a low risk woman who has had a normal delivery and healthy baby home
  after 24 hours, are good things. Deficit-based conversations tend to lock
  us into a 'flatter form/not a flatter form' or a send home/do not send home
  linguistic structure. This is, by its very nature, conservative because it
  confines conversation within this dualism. Words, sentences, images, and
  ideas that lie outside of the dualism tend to be ignored.
- *The silencing of other voices*: Once this kind of conversational dualism
  is established it brings with it another problem. It tends to silence other
  alternative points of view. For example, conversations about male medical

dominance simultaneously serve to reify a distinction between men and women. When conversations about different health care disciplines are couched in the language of turf, territory and conflict, a conversation around difference is sustained. Because the conversation tends to proceed within the terms of the dualism, other realities, values and concerns are removed from earshot.

▨ *The search for deficiencies*: Once locked into the two consequences above, deficit-based conversations are usually sustained by 'type' thinking and a search for certainty and 'truth'. Questions try to expose others and debunk the accounts of those speaking in another way. As a result, conversations with 'others' (other colleagues/staff) tend to slide into an intentional and rigorous search for others' most glaring deficits, deficiencies and weaknesses. Human wholeness and complexity gets lost. The notion of multiple and constructed realities gets lost as well.

▨ *The fragmentation of relationships*: It is no surprise that the posture of those who may, for example, experience deficit-based conversations in their clinical area, is anything other than defensive and disappointed. The energy that is put into reacting to incidents and errors, into trying to minimise risk, to apportion responsibility, blame and so on, only serves to fragment teams and destroy cohesion. It only demoralises and separates. It drives wedges between people rather than bonding them together.

▨ *Negative workplace cultures*: Everything I have said has an impact on workplace cultures. When we have staff who talk in their supervision sessions more about problems than possibilities or more about failures than successes, a culture of negativity can be created. Staff tend to 'close ranks' around preferred ways of talking and interacting. In so doing they re-affirm their relationships, their value positions and their solidarity.

Disclosing aspects of lived experience

A positive question is one that invites staff to reflect upon and then give voice to those aspects of their lived experience (van Manen, 1997) that give them a sense of joy, fulfilment and satisfaction in their work. By asking positive questions, we give ourselves a chance to create powerful vocabularies of possibility, in particular, the possibility of positively re-experiencing past successes and doing more of what satisfies and achieves agreed goals. Through an ethical and appreciative clinical supervision process, the asking of positive questions is habitual. This habit embraces two fundamental concepts of reflection, namely looking back and looking forward: looking back and rediscovering joys, excellence and innovation and looking forward and asking the positive question, 'What single thing, were it to happen again, and more frequently, would make a significant and positive difference to my work here?' When I invite individuals and groups to reflect upon this question, there is usually much discussion around the inclusion of 'and more frequently' and how omitting it from the sentence changes it substantially. Also the phrase 'significant and positive' is a cause of much debate.

How far can clinical supervision be both ethical and appreciative?

If we make the process of clinical supervision ethical and appreciative, we have a chance to:

■ *Release new positive vocabularies.* Positive questions refocus our attention away from problems and towards possibilities. By asking positive questions we invite participants to use words, phrases, sentences and ideas that typically remain uncelebrated or under-used in much of what constitutes normal organisational conversation. This has two consequences. According to Cooperrider (2001: 28):

> First, it begins to loosen the hammerlock that patterns of deficit discourse have on the organisation ... Second, because the restrictive grip of deficit vocabularies is loosened, the positive questions immediately boost energy for action within the organisation. People begin to feel a sense of their own authorship within the organisation. They recognise the strengths and resources that they and others bring to their jobs and this enhances their sense of esteem and efficacy for getting things done. It also generates new ideas for action.

■ *Affirm variety of experience and encourage full voice.* If clinical supervision is about the co-creation of (better) meaning and understanding we are, by implication, adopting a social constructionist view. So it follows that language provides the means through which we communicate the sense we make of our worlds. The language we have available to us, to an extent, determines our possibilities for action. Positive vocabularies give us a chance of acting in the world, positively.

■ *Help us value others even more.* Asking positive questions enables us to appreciate what others value and cherish in their work, and so, understandably, what they want more, not less, of.

■ *Foster relational connections.* Asking a positive question invites those participating in clinical supervision a chance to reflect upon their practice and to think of something significant to them. These are essential things that connect us with others.

■ *Help build a sense of community.* As Cooperrider (2001: 31) says,

> By inviting participants to inquire deeply into the best and most valued aspects of one another's life and work, it immediately creates a context of empathy, care and mutual affirmation.'

Finally, clinical supervision that is both ethical and appreciative enables those involved to grow and evolve in the direction of their most positive guiding images of the future. When supervision sessions are used only as an opportunity to explore misgivings, weaknesses and deficiencies, we gain expert knowledge of what is 'wrong' (or less than desirable) with our own practice, the work of others and our workplace. If supervision is only about this we may become (even) more proficient problem-solvers. By doing this an opportunity is lost to strengthen our collective capacity to imagine and build better services. We miss out on seeing supervision as a process where we create and sustain a culture of possibility and innovation within our health care services.

References:

Anderson H, Gergen K, McNamee S, Cooperrider D, Gergen M, Whitney D (2006) *The Appreciative Organisation*. Chagrin Falls, Taos Institute Publications

Antonacopoulou EP, Gabriel Y (2001) Emotion, learning and organizational change: Towards an integration of psychoanalytic and other perspectives. *J Organizational Change Manag* **14**(5): 435–51

Brookfield S (1994) Tales from the dark side: A phenomenography of adult critical reflection. *Int J Lifelong Edu* **13**(3): 203–16

Carr A (2001) Understanding emotion and emotionality in a process of change. *J Organizational Change Manag* **14**(5): 421–34

Cerney J, Whitney D, Trosten-Bloom A (2004) *Appreciative Team Building: Positive Questions to Bring Out the Best of Your Team*. Illinois, Universe

Cooperrider D (2001) *Working Paper: Appreciative Inquiry: Releasing the Power of the Positive Question*. Case Western Reserve University Cleveland, Ohio. Available online at: http://appreciativeinquiry.case.edu/uploads/working_paper_AI_and_power_positive_question.pdf.

Cooperrider D, Sorensen PF, Yaeger T, Whitney D (eds.) (2005) *Appreciative Inquiry: An Emerging Direction for Organization Development*. Champaign, ILL, Stipes Publishing

Cooperrider D, Whitney D (1999) *Appreciative Inquiry: Collaborating for Change* (booklet). San Francisco, CA, Berrett-Koehler

Cooperrider D, Whitney D (2003) *Appreciative Inquiry Handbook*. San Francisco, CA, Lakeshore Communications and Berrett-Koehler Communications

Cooperrider D, Whitney D (2005) *Appreciative Inquiry: A Positive Revolution in Change*. San Francisco, CA, Berrett-Koehler

De Rivera J (1977) *A Structural Theory of the Emotions*. New York, International Universities Press

Einhorn S (2006) *The Art of Being Kind*. London, Sphere

Gergen K (1994) *Realities and Relationships*. Cambridge, Harvard University Press

Ghaye T (2005) *Developing the Reflective Healthcare Team.* Oxford, Blackwell Publishing

Ghaye T (2007) *Building the Reflective Healthcare Organisation.* Oxford, Blackwell

Hochschild AR (1983) *The Managed Heart: Commercialization of Human Feeling.* Berkeley, CA, University of California Press

Hollway W (1991) *Work Psychology and Organizational Behaviour: Managing the Individual at Work.* London, Sage

Kahane A (2004) *Solving Tough Problems.* San Francisco, CA, Berrett-Koehler

Kolb D, Lublin S, Spoth J, Baker R (1986) Strategic management development using experiential learning theory to assess and develop managerial competencies. *J Manag Development* **5**(3): 13–24

Parry J (2003) Making sense of executive sensemaking: A phenomenological case study with methodological criticism. *J Health Organization Manag* **17**(4): 240–63

Raelin JA (2001) Public reflection as the basis of learning. *Manag Learning* **32**(1): 11–30

Reina D, Reina M (2006) *Trust and Betrayal in the Workplace: Building effective relationships in your organisation.* San Francisco, CA, Berrett-Koehler

Schön D (1983) *The reflective Practitioner: How Professionals Think in Action.* New York, Basic Books

Srivasta S, Cooperrider (eds.) (1990) *Appreciative Leadership and Management. The Power of Positive ?Thought and Action in Organizations.* San Francisco, Jossey-Bass.

Swan E, Bailey A (2004) Thinking with feeling: The emotions of reflection. In: Reynolds M, Vince R (eds) *Organizing Reflection.* Aldershot, Ashgate Publishing

van Manen M (1997) *Researching Lived Experience: Human Science for an Action sensitive Pedagogy.* New York, SUNY Press

Wheatley MJ (2002) *Turning to One Another: Simple Conversations to Restore Hope to the Future.* San Francisco, CA, Berrett-Koehler Publishers

Whitney D, Cooperrider D, Trosten-Bloom A, Kaplin BS (2002) *The Encyclopedia of Positive Questions.* Lakeshore Communications.

Whitney D, Trosten-Bloom A (2002) *The Power of Appreciative Inquiry.* San Francisco, CA, Berrett-Koehler Communications

CHAPTER 3

Implementing clinical supervision within a primary care trust

Debbie Peniket and Sue Lillyman

Introduction

The concept of clinical supervision was identified as a means to ensure safe and accountable practice. The Department of Health, which viewed it as a means of ensuring competence to practice and enhancing consumer protection, defined clinical supervision as

> *A term used to describe a formal process of professional support and learning which enables individual practitioners to develop knowledge and competence, assume responsibility for their own practice and enhance consumer protection and safety of care in a complex clinical situation ... and should be seen as a means of encouraging assessment, analytical and reflective skills.*
>
> Department of Health (1993: 15)

In the document *Making a Difference* (Department of Health, 1999) clinical supervision is also seen as integral to an organisation's clinical governance strategy which, according to Lipp and Osbourne (2000) actively promotes the clinical governance agenda. The importance of clinical supervision was again reinforced in the *National Policy Agenda, NHS Plan* (Department of Health, 2000). These documents highlight that clinical supervision has now become an established part of the working practice of many nurses and allied health professionals (AHPs). As Burton (2000) points out it has now become part of continuing professional development and it is therefore unlikely to be displaced. These documents also identify that the strength of the NHS is in its staff and the need to support and develop its staff to meet the daily challenges is reinforced by the need for continuity of quality improvement.

The benefit of clinical supervision was also noted by Driscoll (2000) who suggested that patients experienced a certain type of care from practitioners engaged in clinical supervision. Timpson (1996) and Wray *et al* (1998) also noted an increase in the quality of patient care.

The Primary Care Trust

South Birmingham Primary Care Trust (PCT) came into being in April 2002. At that time it was the largest PCT in England serving a population of 383 000. The population characteristics present the PCT with key public health issues and in addition it is a complex organisation with a significant commissioning role and a large service provider function including specialist services that are provided on a city and region-wide basis.

There are approximately 3000 staff directly employed in the PCT. Of these 1850 are nurses, health visitors, AHPs, clinical scientists, clinical technologists, technicians and support staff such as rehabilitation assistants. There are an additional 95 practice nurses employed by general practitioners. This group of staff, who comprise 60% of the workforce, have a huge impact on the ability of the PCT to deliver the NHS Plan through the service improvement agenda.

The development of the South Birmingham PCT Strategy for Nursing, Therapy and Health Care Science in 2003 provided a framework within which staff could be recruited, developed and supported in delivering excellence in clinical practice to ensure quality improvements in patient care. This strategy acknowledged the importance of clinical supervision both in achieving this and in nurturing a culture of support, reflection and learning. A framework and action plan was therefore developed as a follow on to the strategy in order to support the implementation of clinical supervision across the PCT. One of the differences with this framework is that it recognises that all staff benefit from support, reflection and personal development. Therefore it not only relates to clinical staff on the wards or in clinical practice but also includes both clinical and non-clinical staff working within the trust.

The action plan to support implementation included:

- The setting up of a steering group to develop further the framework, to oversee implementation and to monitor and report on progress.
- The setting up of a 'pilot project' with community staff selected because the nature of their work often means they work in isolation in a very demanding area of the city.
- The completion of a staff survey.
- The arrangement of an 'event' to share models in use across the trust and look at options for taking them forward.
- The visiting of all directorates in order to establish what was needed at directorate level in terms of training and support.
- The provision of a trust-wide training programme.
- The setting up of an internet web page to support staff seeking supervision and to provide a network for staff.

The Steering Group

A steering group was formed from all directorates across the trust ensuring a multidisciplinary team approach. The Assistant Director of Nursing and therapies provided leadership in partnership with a senior lecturer from a local university who had an interest and expertise in this subject. The Steering Group met monthly and one of the first discussions included the topic of clinical supervision. Although the term is well accepted within nursing through the Nursing and Midwifery Council's position papers (Nursing and Midwifery Council, 2000) some professional groups and non-clinical staff felt that it might cause practitioners to misinterpret the process. The title 'supervision' implied a managerial approach and 'clinical' suggested that it related only to nursing or allied health professionals. Clinical supervision can have the potential to constitute a form of surveillance according to Clouder and Sellars (2004) and so to break down this barrier, and not confuse the process with managerial supervision, the title of 'practice support' was adopted. This had already been used within the trust and conveyed the message of a non-managerial approach and the giving of support to staff. The group then developed its own definition of what practice support meant, stating that,

> *Practice support enables staff to discuss their work on a regular basis with other experienced individuals. The process will enable staff to seek support, provide the opportunity to reflect and learn from their practice, develop skills and competence in their work and enhance patient care.*
>
> (South Birmingham Primary Care Trust, 2006)

The Steering Group had a key role in facilitating and supporting the implementation process. It also provided the overview, progress reports and assurance to the senior management team and the clinical governance committee.

Developing the framework 'Practice Support for All'

The framework supports the need for continuous quality improvement and personal development. It recognises that the strength of the PCT is in its staff, whose skills, expertise and dedication underpin the delivery of care. It highlights the trust's commitment to assist all staff in accessing practice support while recognising the individual's own responsibility for personal development.

The framework was developed within the trust, with acknowledgements to a local acute trust which had previously developed its framework and provided help with the contents. At each stage of the framework development it was returned to the Steering Group for comments and once completed, it was presented at both the Professional Executive Committee and the Clinical Governance Committee for approval.

The Steering Group, as stated, included representatives from all the directorates within the PCT and as such had a wealth of experience in the need for, and delivery of, clinical supervision. Many of the directorates had pockets of practice support and clinical supervision in progress and the intention was not to change any of the good practice in place, but to assist those areas that had not been exposed to the process and help those that had not undertaken it before.

The framework needed to remain flexible to incorporate existing good practice within the trust, and not be too prescriptive in relation to the models of clinical supervision, practice support or reflective practice that could be used. Practitioners were also encouraged to choose the option of one-to-one, group, network or team supervision according to their needs.

Documentation of the session caused debate among Steering Group members. Although it was agreed that the contents of the session were confidential, for audit purposes the trust would need to know how many members of staff were receiving supervision and the frequency and duration of the supervision sessions. A form was included for participants to complete (see *Figure 3.1*) and would be used in relation to fulfilling the clinical governance agenda.

The relationship between clinical governance and clinical supervision has been emphasised by Butterworth and Woods who proposed that:

Participating in clinical supervision in an active way is a demonstration of an individual exercising his or her responsibility under clinical governance and that clinical supervision should be seen as an integral part of a framework of activities that are designed to manage, enhance and monitor delivery of high quality services.

Butterworth and Woods (1998)

This has subsequently been reinforced in the publication of the Healthcare Commission's *Standards for Better Health* (Department of Health, 2004).

Reflective practice in the clinical supervision session

Reflective practice and clinical supervision are not synonymous although reflective practice is integral to the process and purpose of clinical supervision (Heath and Freshwater, 2000; Lipp, 2001). Reflection is also a prerequisite for all practitioners (Chartered Society of Physiotherapy, 2000; Nursing and Midwifery Council, 2002, 2004). Supervisees are encouraged to maintain

---

Record of meeting

Name of supervisor ....,

Date .... Time ....

Duration... Venue ....

Names of those attending (supervisees or group members):

....

....

....

Outside speaker invited:

....

Comments:

....

....

....

....

Date and time of next meeting: ....

Figure 3.1. Record of meeting.

their own reflective records of the session to keep within their own personal development records and portfolios. This is encouraged in the framework and an example is provided in *Figure 3.2*. The practitioner completes each section and keeps the record in a safe place. It is envisaged that this reflection will lead practitioners to new insights within their own practice. Recorded accounts will also assist practitioners to gain evidence for their knowledge and skills requirements as well as professional portfolios.

What does practice support (clinical supervision) mean?

The benefits and purpose of practice support were summed up in the framework as:

▪ Improvement of clinical standards and quality of patient care. The was the central purpose (Timpson, 1996; Butterworth and Woods, 1998; Wray *et al*, 1998; Hansbo and Kihlgren, 2004).

Reflective record

This is confidential to the supervisee(s) and should be recorded and kept as part of their personal portfolio.

Issue(s) discussed (Key Skills Framework Domain):

....

Key issues identified from the discussions:

....

Areas identified for personal research/reading and/or knowledge development:

....

Areas where new knowledge/skills/attitudes identified within the session:

....

Learning point:

....

Personal action plan for future practice:

....

Figure 3.2. A reflective record.

- Increased feeling of support and feelings of possible personal well-being (Butterworth *et al*, 1996; Kirkham and Stapleton, 2000).
- Increased confidence and decreased incidence of emotional strain (Berg and Hallberg, 1999).
- Higher staff morale and satisfaction leading to decrease in staff sickness/ absence and increased staff satisfaction (Butterworth *et al*, 1996).
- Learning through difficult experiences and engaging in reflective practice (Johns, 2004).
- Increased self-awareness (Cutliffe and Epling, 1997).

It should not be viewed as 'confessional' practice (Clouder and Sellars, 2004). Butterworth (1992) and Cutcliffe and Proctor (1998) also alluded to the problems that would ensue if clinical supervision were blended and fused together with managerial supervision. However Kirkham and Stapleton (2000) found in their study that the need to support through listening, 'off loading' and someone who would be there in the supportive capacity was the best form of supervision.

The staff survey

A survey was undertaken to identify where clinical supervision was established and working well in the trust. Staff were then invited to present and share their good practice at a half-day event. The survey was sent out to 25% ($n = 958$) of the workforce across the trust with a return of 218 questionnaires. The findings identified a positive approach to clinical supervision although some staff were unsure what constituted clinical supervision at present and were confused with the Individual Performance Review and other forms of supervision.

The survey identified that all staff were already receiving some type of supervision in their practice although this included performance review and other managerial processes. Eighty-nine staff were supervising staff internally with another six supervising other professionals externally. Of the 218 who returned their questionnaires 102 had received some form of training and only one found this unhelpful. Clinical supervision was considered a good idea by 201.

The pilot project

Discussions were held with staff and managers in community services to determine the benefits of setting up a pilot project for the implementation of clinical supervision with a team of staff who were experiencing demanding caseloads in terms of social deprivation, child protection, domestic violence and drug abuse. The team included health visitors, a school nurse, a nursery nurse, a link worker and an administrator. Supervision was being accessed in relation to specific child protection cases, but not in relation to other aspects of their role.

Training, support and facilitation were offered to the team and a model of group clinical supervision was agreed to try and deliver the outcomes that the team identified as being beneficial to them. These included:

- A lessening of feelings of isolation.
- An increase in the levels of support.
- An improvement in communication among members of the team.
- The development of strategies for coping with the demands that came with working in this difficult environment.

The chocolate orange model

The Assistant Director of Nursing and Therapies who was leading this process had previously received training in clinical supervision when working in a clinical role. The training was delivered to established clinical teams and had encouraged these teams to develop their own model. The model presented here was developed by a team of clinicians specialising in the rehabilitation of patients with acquired brain injury, and was presented to the pilot group to illustrate the concept and potential benefits if adapted to their own situation and needs. The model was known as the Chocolate Orange Model of Clinical Support and is presented with acknowledgements to former colleagues in the Rehabilitation Directorate of the PCT.

Protocol and ground rules

Definition

Clinical support is a structured, supportive, interactive process that encourages health care professionals to take protected time out in a safe, trusting environment to exchange and facilitate reflective discussions.

Aim

Clinical support aims to facilitate reflection on practice and feelings about work, in order to learn from experience and continuously improve competence and the patient and staff experience.

Model

The Chocolate Orange Model of Clinical Support is an all encompassing model (*Figure 3.3*) that acknowledges that clinical support is a process that is placed within an organisational context (box), requires a supportive, safe environment in which to take place (wrapper), and comprises several components (segments) that together achieve continuing personal and professional development for the individual and results in beneficial outcomes to the service user.

Method

Group support had been chosen on its merits. Its advantages and disadvantages are outlined in *Table 3.1*. The number in the group ranged from four to six with the roles of reflective learner, facilitator and administrator rotating within the session. The administrator is the person who attends to the management of the meeting such as time keeping, sticking to the subject under discussion, and adhering to the ground rules. The meetings were held monthly and each member was encouraged to present an 'issue' at each practice support session. A maximum of 30 minutes per member was allowed with a maximum meeting time of three hours and an anticipated minimum time of two hours.

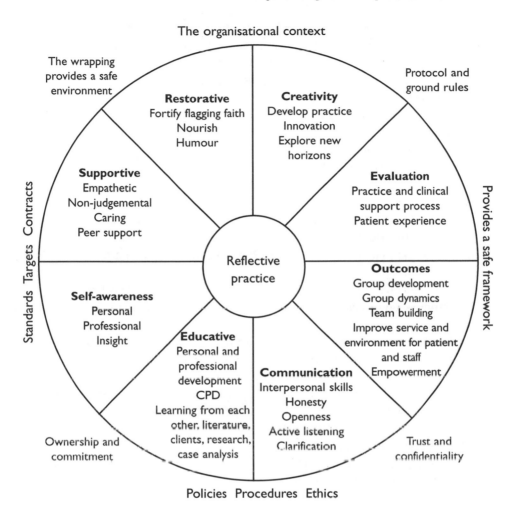

Figure 3.3. The Chocolate Orange Model of Clinical Support. CPD: continuing professional development.

Location

The location requirements are:

- Away from the clinical area but on site.
- Reserved room (with drinks facilities).
- Confidential environment.
- Informal seating arrangement.
- Meeting in progress sign to be used.
- No telephones in the room.
- Mobile phones to be switched off.

Table 3.1. Advantages and disadvantages of group support

Advantages	*Disadvantages*
▪ Provides a setting where problems can be worked on by the whole group, every member is a potential helper	▪ No space for a focus 'just on me' without a group spotlight
▪ Participants gain from hearing about critical incidents, from both different and similar to their own experience	▪ Confidentiality is more difficult to maintain
	▪ Individuals get less time
▪ Several different perspectives may emerge on any issue	▪ One person may dominate
	▪ Some people may be less likely to disclose personal issues
▪ Participants can provide restorative mutual support	▪ The most reflective people of all may be less inclined to contribute
▪ Participants will be empowered by group support	▪ Supervisors need group work skills in addition to supervision skills
▪ Participants who set up and facilitate groups can benefit from experiencing and reflecting on the group processes involved	
▪ It is time efficient	

Timing

It was agreed that the group would decide on a regular time for the meeting and this time would be identified as protected time and so should avoid regular commitments such as clinics.

Content of session

A 'preview' of all group members' issues would be given before starting, to prioritise time. and a chocolate grading system would assist with prioritisation:

1.   White   Low
2.   Milk |
3.   Dark |
4.   Fondue!!   Crisis

The sessions would be flexible according to needs and agreed by members of the group. An action plan/points would be set with the agreement of the group and an opportunity for reflection on the session would be provided at the end.

Documentation

It was agreed that each member would keep a notebook or diary in which to record that the meeting took place, its duration and a note of who had attended. The reflective learner was given the right of veto over note taking and topics discussed could be reviewed within the group at 6 monthly intervals to identify recurring themes as part of the evaluation process.

Roles and responsibilities of a reflective learner and facilitator

The roles and responsibilities of a reflective learner and facilitator are shown in *Table 3.2*.

Confidentiality

Complete confidentiality must be maintained and the group should decide if issues can be divulged outside of the forum. Conversations and ideas should not be quoted or sourced, neither should it be reported who or what was said.

If unsafe practice (ie. a situation where a patient could have come to harm or has come to harm) or bad practice (ie. where a patient has experienced a near miss) is demonstrated, confidentialities may need to be broken. If unsafe practice has already been reported to managers, further action need not be taken. The group will maintain a supportive forum for those involved.

Training

It is recommended that, before joining the group, new members should have some training, to include communication and group work skills. In addition new members will be required to read the protocol, ground rules and be aware of the model.

Table 3.2. Roles and responsibilities of reflective learner and facilitator

Reflective learner	Joint responsibilities	Facilitator
Reflect	Confidentiality	Guide
Identify and own issues and agenda	Sharing information	Active listening and constructive feedback
Respond to feedback	Contributing to a safe environment	
		Supportive
	Identifying trends – personal/service/clinical	Exploratory and raising awareness
	Defining relationship	
		Empathy
	Honest and open	
		Non-judgemental
	Positive, valuable experience	
	Willingness for participation	

Grievance procedure

This may be referred to if confidentiality is broken or if protocol or ground rules are breached.

Evaluation

A review of the entire process and outcomes should take place after six months. This review should be by discussion in the group and by use of an audit tool. The protocol should be reviewed and revised annually although it may be reviewed earlier if agreed by the group.

Contract

All group members should sign the contract and if new members join, the contract should be re-signed by all members.

The above process was adopted by the pilot group with some adaptations. They referred to their process as group practice support and it was inclusive of clinical and non-clinical members. Facilitation was provided initially by a senior lecturer from the local university with a plan to hand this back to the group once confidence in the process was established.

Evaluating the project

After a six-month period the pilot group was asked to evaluate the meetings. One of the main issues raised was that the professional group with the most members, in this instance health visitors, tended to dominate the subject being discussed. It was felt that time was an issue and often problems arose from managers in relation to time spent at the meeting and the measurable benefit to the workplace. Although finding time for attendance was difficult most members of the team felt that it was important to spend time together and work through work-related issues. It was agreed that all members attend the first half hour but the health visitors would continue with issues that related specifically to their work therefore utilising the time more effectively for other group members.

Positive aspects included the group having the opportunity to meet together as they often felt isolated in their current practice. The meetings also enhanced communication and better understanding of each other's workload. Group members were able to share knowledge and felt more of a team being able to meet to discuss both issues of concern and good practice. This was preferable to managerial meetings with set agendas.

Summary

Once an organisation has decided to implement clinical supervision, and has invested in training, actual implementation is a lengthy process (Winstanley and White, 2002).

Variations in the structure and process of clinical supervision have occurred largely as a result of local policy and managerial decisions made within each organisation about how to integrate clinical supervision into working practice. Even within an overall positive disposition toward clinical supervision, several difficulties have been reported. Finding time for clinical supervision sessions was principal among these and this was particularly so in practice settings where the usefulness of clinical supervision was doubted. Elsewhere, resistance from clinicians is reported and those who needed supervision the most were those least likely to attend sessions or to facilitate the attendance of others. In the survey of staff working within South Birmingham PCT, many noted time as a problem and lack of management structure was also an issue.

Clinical supervision in South Birmingham had evolved in line with the national picture. It had developed in pockets and there were a variety of models in place. The approach outlined in this chapter is facilitating progress towards consistent involvement in a process (practice support) that embraces the principles of clinical supervision but that also emphasises the supportive aspect and is inclusive of all staff.

References

Berg A, Hallberg IR (1999) Effects of systematic clinical supervision on psychiatric nurses' sense of coherent, creativity, work-related strain, job satisfaction and view of the effects from clinical supervision: A pre-post test design. *J Psych Ment Health Nurs* **6**: 371–81

Burton S (2000) A critical essay on professional development in dietetics through a process of reflection and clinical supervision. *J Human Nutr Dietetics* **5**: 317–22

Butterworth T (1992) Clinical supervision as an emerging idea in nursing. In Butterworth T, Faugier J (eds) *Clinical Supervision and Mentorship in Nursing.* London, Chapman Hall

Butterworth T, Bishop V, Carson J (1996) First steps towards evaluating clinical supervision in nursing and health visiting: Theory, policy and practice development. *Rev J Clin Nurs* **5**: 127–32

Butterworth T, Woods D (1998) *Clinical Governance and Clinical Supervision: Working Together to Ensure Safe and Accountable Practice – A Briefing Paper.* Manchester: University of Manchester

Chartered Society of Physiotherapy (2000) *Clinical Supervision – Information Paper PA 45.* London, Chartered Society of Physiotherapy

Clouder L, Sellars J (2004) Reflective practice and clinical supervision: An interprofessional perspective. *J Adv Nurs* **46**(3): 262–9

Cutcliffe RJ, Epling M (1997) An exploration of the use of John Heron's confronting interventions in clinical supervision: Case studies from practice. *Psych Care* **4**(1): 174–80

Cutcliffe RJ, Proctor B (1998) An alternative training approach to clinical supervision. *Br J Nurs* **7**(5): 280–5

Driscoll J (2000) *Practising Clinical Supervision: A Reflective Approach.* London, Bailliere Tindall

Department of Health (1993) *Vision for the Future.* London, Department of Health

Department of Health (1999) *Making a Difference.* London, Department of Health

epartment of Health (2000) *Meeting the Challenge, A Strategy for Allied Health Professionals.* London, Department of Health

Department of Health (2004) *Standards for Better Health.* London, Department of Health

Hansebo G, Kihlgren M (2004) Nursing home care: Changes after supervision. *J Adv Nurs* **45**(3): 269–79

Heath H, Freshwater D (2000) Clinical supervision as an emancipatory process: Avoiding inappropriate intent. *J Adv Nurs* **32**: 1298–306

Johns C (2004) *Becoming a Reflective Practitioner* (2nd edn). Oxford, Blackwell Publications

Kirkham M, Stapleton H (2000) Midwives' Support Needs as Childbirth Changes. *J Adv Nurs* **32**(2): 465–72

Lipp A (2001) Clinical supervision as part of clinical governance. An instrument of oppression or liberation. *J Clin Excellence* **2**: 203–7

Lipp A, Osborne P (2000) Clinical supervision and clinical governance: The art and science of bridge building. *J Clin Excellence* **2**(1): 3–8

Nursing and Midwifery Council (2000) *Position Statement on Clinical Supervision for Nurses and Health Visitors*. London, Nursing and Midwifery Council

Nursing and Midwifery Council (2002) *Supporting Nurses and Midwives Through Life Long Learning*. London, Nursing and Midwifery Council

Nursing and Midwifery Council (2004) *The PREP Handbook*. London, Nursing and Midwifery Council

South Birmingham Primary Care Trust (2006) *Practice Support (Clinical Supervision) for All. A Framework for South Birmingham Primary Care Trust*. Birmingham, South Birmingham Primary Care Trust

Timpson J (1996) Clinical supervision: A plan for 'pit head time' in cancer nursing. *Eur J Cancer Nurs* **5**(1): 42–52

Wray F, Ferguson M, Hudson N (1998) A sharing, caring experience. *Paediatr Nurs* **10**(9): 6–8

Winstanley J, White E (2002) Clinical Supervision: Models, measures and best practice. *Nurse Researcher* **10**(4): 7–38

CHAPTER 4

Challenges for student nurses requiring clinical supervision

Karen Latimer

Introduction

The primary aim of my research was to demonstrate the barriers facing student nurses requiring clinical supervision. The study showed how student nurses benefit from regular clinical supervision if it is incorporated within the pre-registration curriculum. This can then become a vehicle for sustaining supervision, once the student nurse has made the transition to newly qualified staff nurse. The study also highlighted a deficit in the provision of clinical supervision within a majority of diploma in higher education pre-registration programmes across Britain for student nurses. In order to identify the deficit of clinical supervision within these programmes, a survey was undertaken of how many universities within Britain provide clinical supervision within their diploma and degree pre-registration curricula.

Background of the study

The clinical facilitator's role (Department of Health, 1999; Rowan and Barber, 2000) is to work with students and their mentors within their placement areas so as to assist with the acquisition of knowledge and skills. Clinical facilitators provide clinical skills study days to help students practise skills before they are formally assessed and undertake these skills within the placement area. Therefore, the clinical facilitator is ideally positioned to promote the concept of clinical supervision, while utilising a reflective practice model (Schön, 1987).

When exploring the research question of whether or not student nurses require clinical supervision it was already being provided to students within their placement areas on a one-to-one basis. It was then introduced at clinical skills days to groups of student nurses at various stages within their training. Feedback both verbally and from written evaluation forms clearly showed that student nurses found the clinical supervision sessions very beneficial. In addition, they also stated how the sessions had begun to increase their confidence and their performance within their nursing practice. This was not a new phenomenon. During previous experience as a professional development nurse supporting both newly qualified staff nurses and senior nurses, part of the role had been the responsibility to provide regular clinical supervision on both a one-to-one and group basis. From this experience of having conducted numerous sessions, feedback had nearly always been positive. However, while working as a clinical facilitator it was evident that student nurses were not receiving the same opportunities as their post-registration colleagues in access to clinical supervision. This was an important oversight that needed to be addressed. It was at this point that I then began to look more closely at the university's pre-registration curriculum, to find out whether or not the nursing tutors were providing clinical supervision for their students. Nursing journals were scanned to discover whether others had reported this perceived deficit within student nurse training or whether it was just a local problem. It was decided that part of the research would require networking (Vaughan, 1996) with other universities, to explore whether or not they provided clinical supervision within their pre-registration programmes.

Identifying the sample

The participants involved in the study were principally student nurses in the third year of training. It was the intention to find out how student nurses felt about receiving supervision through the different stages of their training and how they would perceive continuing this model once they were qualified staff nurses. In addition, 50 universities were surveyed in relation to the inclusion or omission of clinical supervision within their degree and diploma pre-registration programmes.

Using a phenomenological/action research approach

A phenomenological approach was adopted, with the inquiry being managed through the use of action research. A phenomenological approach aims to promote an understanding of the human experience from an individual researcher's perspective (Cormack, 2002). This approach also enabled access to the effects of emotional, social and physical well-being of the student nurses, which would be important in relation to the concept of clinical supervision being embraced and taken forward as a positive development in their future career progression.

It was also decided to use elements of action research, because the student nurses were moving through their training and, as Cormack (2002) points out, action research involves the researcher working with research participants to analyse the situation they want to change and to plan how to change it. In addition, action research also involves a change intervention, which aims at improvement and involvement. Furthermore, it involves a cyclic process in which research, action and evaluation are interlinked (Blaxter *et al*, 2002). The plan was to follow the students' development, being mindful that time would be limited due to the 12-month time-scale allocated for this particular study. I was ideally placed to undertake action research because of being within the situation and the organisation in which the students undertook their practice. According to Robson (2002) the researcher's position within the research process is significant, because ideally the researcher should be part of the development, which is viewed as a pre-requisite for undertaking a method such as action research.

Collecting the data

The research design generated both quantitative and qualitative data, and the variety of data-gathering methods that were utilised added validity through triangulation.

A qualitative approach was employed with the aim of understanding the experience of the participant (Blaxter, 1996). Qualitative research is a systematic, subjective approach used to describe life experiences and situations to give them meaning, in phenomenological terms, to capture the 'lived experience' of the study participants (Burns and Grove, 2003). This was relevant and in context with the students' situation so questionnaires were used to obtain the information that was required. The participants chosen to receive questionnaires were in their third year of training and were in their last six months of their programme. Robson (2002) refers to this as purposive sampling, as this typically involves researchers using their judgement to achieve a particular purpose. The group was purposely chosen because firstly, they had previously received 12 months of clinical supervision either on a one-to-one or group basis with sessions between one month and six weeks apart. Secondly, this group was due to qualify as staff nurses in the near future, which meant that their answers on how to continue supervision once they were qualified was relevant.

A quantitative approach was also used to collect and analyse data in a numeric form. These data consisted of information obtained from the universities which were surveyed, that incorporated clinical supervision within both their degree and diploma pre-registration programmes. Telephone interviews and email were used to obtain information regarding the inclusion of clinical supervision from 50 universities nationwide (Robson, 2002).

Findings of the study

The results of the study were twofold. The expected findings of the proposed research identified the impact of clinical supervision on both the student nurses' clinical practice and professional development. In addition, the data also determined what barriers exist (if any) to the implementation of clinical supervision for student nurses and identified strategies that would enable them to take forward the process of clinical supervision once they were qualified. A survey of the universities also revealed that there was a lack of consistency between the diploma pre-registration curricula nationally, in terms of the interpretation of clinical supervision, and its relationship with reflective practice. The results of this study are discussed in light of previous published literature concerning clinical supervision.

The overall responses to the clinical supervision questionnaire yielded very positive results. The students were asked to rate how valuable clinical supervision was for their clinical practice and professional development. The responses were positive and supported by previous literature (Nicklin, 1995; Butterworth *et al*, 1996; United Kingdom Central Council, 1996; Goorapah, 1997; Severinsson and Borgenhammer, 1997; Webb, 1997; Bishop, 1998; Dunn, 1999; Jones, 1999). The barriers the student nurses identified are also acknowledged in the literature review, with time constraints being one of the major factors (May, 2003). The lack of time available to carry out clinical supervision is also discussed by Marrow *et al* (1998) who agree that it requires support and commitment by organisations because of resource implications. The research focused the student nurses on how they would ensure clinical supervision was continued when they qualified as staff nurses. All of the students appeared to be united on specific strategies such as asking for details about it at interviews for staff nurse posts within the trust, discussing it with their managers, finding out who the clinical supervisors were within the trust and finally discussing with their colleagues about what was available within the trust.

This information was useful because the responses to the questions relating to both the barriers that existed and what strategies they would use to ensure the continuation of clinical supervision on qualifying would form the basis of an action plan. The aim was to disseminate this information to the clinical trainer within the trust. The clinical trainer supports newly qualified staff nurses through a preceptorship programme (Myrick, 2002), and this information would ensure the continuation of clinical supervision. If organisations were to place a higher value on nursing staff receiving regular supervision, student nurses and newly qualified nurses would then view supervision as a natural progression, and ensure that it became a part of everyday nursing practice.

Clinical supervision within the curriculum

The evidence from the universities indicated inconsistencies in the provision of clinical supervision, especially between the diploma and degree courses. The large numbers of students within the diploma nursing programmes meant that neither one-to-one nor group supervision could be facilitated. One reason given was lack of time due to other work commitments, which reflects issues surrounding time constraints (May, 2003). Another reason was that it was not possible to maintain the sessions once the students were in clinical practice, again due to other work commitments. This confirms Murray's (2001) findings in relation to overstretched lecturers. Also reported was a lack of clinical facilitators within the trust, with some lecturers stating that they believed clinical supervision to be 'very similar to reflection', and 'we already get our students to sometimes reflect on critical incidents in their personal tutorials'.

In addition, further comments included, 'there was no point because the qualified staff nurses were not undertaking clinical supervision within the trust anyway' and 'there is already a shortage of qualified staff nurses within the clinical areas, and clinical supervision may add to their clinical workloads'. These practical issues appeared to discourage the lecturers from providing any supervision due to the fact that it would not be continued once the students were in clinical practice. This is also reflected within the literature (Scanlon and Weir, 1997; Durrai and Kendrick, 1999; Price and Chalker, 2000). However, all the universities did say that they encouraged their students to use personal reflective diaries and to include reflection within their assignments. In contrast, the degree programmes, which had smaller student numbers, managed to provide clinical supervision and embraced the concept more fully as sound professional practice.

Reflection and clinical supervision

The point about reflection and clinical supervision being viewed differently was highlighted. Inskipp and Proctor (1993), Bishop (1994) and Jones (1996) all insist that reflection and supervision are intrinsically linked. However, this now appears to be questionable. The impact of having large student groups in the diploma programmes with the added pressure of not always having clinical facilitators within the trusts did seem to have contributed to the separation of clinical supervision and reflective practice.

It could be argued, however, that student nurses could be receiving clinical supervision while having personal tutor support, as all the universities did provide each student with a personal tutor. Although tutorials may not be recognised as a formal mechanism for clinical supervision, they do provide an ideal opportunity for one-to-one clinical supervision, because personal tutorial support is undertaken in a safe, confidential environment (Butterworth, 1997; May, 2003). Williams (2001) supports the view that nurse education needs to undertake a key role in helping students develop their skills of reflection. It would perhaps be possible for the personal tutor to encompass clinical supervision by formalising the process of reflection. Although, as Murray

(2001) points out, nurse lecturers are already overstretched and, with the high numbers of diploma nursing students, this may not be feasible.

Should clinical supervision be mandatory in pre-registration courses?

Overall clinical supervision does not seem to appear on the pre-registration national curriculum, and in addition, it also appears that there are only pockets of good practice within a few universities and hospital trusts nationwide. Another dimension to the provision of clinical supervision is whom would most benefit? As May (2003: 61) states, 'clinical supervision is an essential tool in the continuing development of all nurses, whether newly qualified or at senior level'. If clinical supervision were to be introduced within pre-registration training and became mandatory, this could provide the answer for post-registered nurses. It is possible that these nurses may then feel empowered to take ownership for themselves, and help motivate them to take positive steps to ensure that their current employers provide opportunities for supervision to take place. As May continues, 'employers should provide protected supervision time for nurses – in itself a demonstration that practitioners are valued and trusted to use this time effectively'. Butterworth *et al* (1996) support May's viewpoint and add that employers would not only be supporting nursing staff but also enhancing patient care. This is because, 'as supervised nurses they are more likely to reflect on patient need and the associated practice dilemmas, thereby ensuring best practice and professional development' (May, 2003: 61).

It is this evidence that strengthens the belief in the effectiveness of reflective practice through clinical supervision (Schön, 1987; Bright 1995; Butterworth, 1997) and how valuable its implementation would be for student nurses.

Cultural changes needed for clinical supervision

As previously stated, this study formed the basis for demonstrating that pre-registration student nurses benefit from regular clinical supervision, which could be the vehicle for sustaining supervision once the student nurse qualifies. From the results of the study it is clear that certain implications for practice exist for the student nurses, the hospital trust and the university. Further research and exploration is needed into incorporating clinical supervision early on within the pre-registration programme with a possible focus on cultural changes within organisations such as universities and the NHS, so that they recognise the value of the concept and are committed to the provision of clinical supervision for all professionals, not only nurses. Bishop (1998), Lowry (1998) and Donaldson (2001) have all commented on the way in which nursing is practised. Cultural changes require a change in traditional work patterns and routines; clinical governance is viewed as the framework to support these changes by developing leadership and management skills. This would aim to provide a top down approach, which may be required for nurses so that they are empowered and are able to take ownership of clinical supervision. As Pursey (1995) says, clinical supervision needs to be supported from the top of the organisation and defined from the bottom. It requires resources, commitment and a collective vision.

Preparing students to achieve appropriate competency

Reflective practice is seen as a major part of curriculum activity, but the style in which reflection is advocated is not necessarily clinical supervision. May (2003) supports the view that clinical supervision should be protected time for nurses, with it being an essential process in the continuing development of all nurses. As May (2003: 2) states, 'students are supported in a non-threatening environment to discuss practice issues and, through this process, are able to identify their strengths and weaknesses and improve their communication skills.' Ajiboye (2000) says that supporting students on their clinical placements to achieve the appropriate levels of competency can be undertaken by a mentor, facilitator or assessor. Consistent clinical supervision in a supportive learning environment is fundamental to the student's success (Ajiboye, 2000; May, 2003). Ajiboye (2000: 53) takes this point further stating 'in line with the NHS Plan (Department of Health, 2000), students of today will be expected to take centre stage tomorrow, in delivering optimum health care as highly competent and reflective practitioners, capable of making crucial decisions.'

Developing the curriculum

If clinical supervision is not incorporated and implemented within the curriculum, an opportunity will be missed. The literature supports the impact and perceived benefits of clinical supervision, benefits that could be enjoyed by both individual practitioners, the NHS and patients/clients. By not introducing and sustaining clinical supervision within nursing universally, it would appear to contradict what other professions, such as midwifery, counselling, social work and mental health care, have in place (Hawkins and Shohet, 1989; Durrai and Kendrick, 1999). In addition, other countries, such as the USA, Sweden, Australia, Canada, South Africa and Slovenia, all currently promote reflective practice or clinical supervision within their student nurse training programmes (Antonsson and Sandstroem, 2000; Kok and Chabeli, 2002; Lepp *et al*, 2003).

There is a lack of consistency between the universities that deliver the pre-registration curriculum and it would be desirable to standardise the way in which the curriculum is interpreted and developed to include clinical supervision for both degree and diploma nursing students to ensure equity and parity. There have already been modifications in nursing curricula, mainly in the degree programmes, which are currently encompassing an alignment towards clinical supervision (Jones, 1999). A multi-faceted approach would ensure that clinical supervision could be sustained using systems that already exist such as clinical facilitators within trusts and personal tutors within universities.

Role of clinical trainers

Information from this study would essentially form an important part of the clinical trainer's strategy for implementing clinical supervision for this group of staff. This preliminary groundwork also means that clinical trainers could now develop a robust strategy to take forward clinical supervision for newly qualified nurses. In fact, this is another aspect of the research already undertaken which could be extended and explored further, especially in terms of how successful the strategy was in its implementation and how useful the information gained from this study has been for both clinical trainers and newly qualified staff nurses. Johns and Freshwater (1998: 166) add, 'the processes of action research, clinical supervision and reflective practice complement each other in bringing together theory and research in an attempt to challenge previous practice.'

Conclusions

It can be concluded that clinical supervision for pre-registration students could be the vehicle for sustaining aspects such as life-long learning and continuing professional development, once the student nurse has qualified. Whatever the impetus behind the process of clinical supervision, the suggestion from the majority of the literature is that clinical supervision will help to solve a variety of problems including management issues, standards of patient care, professional development, staff stress and workforce morale. If any of these are to be achieved, the experiences outlined in the literature indicate there are a variety of barriers to overcome in order to implement effective clinical supervision (Bishop, 1998; May, 2003). The primary purpose of this research was to enable pre-registration student nurses to benefit from regular clinical supervision which would assist them with sustaining supervision once they qualify as staff nurses.

The literature failed to echo this viewpoint because, as previously stated, there appear to be extensive gaps in terms of clinical supervision being essential for student nurses and regarding the continuation of supervision once the students have qualified. Although the literature does confirm the need for protected time for nursing staff, it does not suggest how this can be achieved (May, 2003). A possible solution which Lowry (1998) and Cairns (1998) propose, is that the Nursing and Midwifery Council (2002) ensures that clinical supervision is made a mandatory requirement for all registered nurses. This would then perhaps have the desired effect of ensuring that clinical supervision is incorporated within pre-registration programmes routinely because it is viewed as a part of everyday practice for nurses. The results of this study confirmed that student nurses could take control of their own development by selecting appropriate strategies to assist them with taking clinical supervision forward to when they qualified.

Limitation of the study

The research limitation identified was the need for a further study to assess whether or not clinical supervision could be sustained when student nurses qualified.

This research cannot be heralded as conclusive proof that clinical supervision results in maintaining standards, enhancing professional development and reducing stress and burnout. However, I believe it provides a significant contribution to how both the NHS trusts and universities could provide opportunities for student nurses to receive clinical supervision both during their pre-registration training and on qualification, with the outcomes of improved morale and job satisfaction and enriched nursing practice. Through the facilitation of clinical supervision, nurses become empowered and are able to value their interactions as a therapeutic resource. With more time and greater resources, it may have been beneficial to extend the study over three years. This would have allowed comparisons to be drawn between the different groups at the various stages of their training programme.

Personal reflections

Personally, reflecting on the research process has been beneficial in terms of developing critical thinking as a researcher. Fisher (1996) describes reflection as an opportunity to look back and discuss experiences, which focuses on thoughts and feelings, as the reflector moves through the process. Johns and Freshwater (1998: 2) concur, 'through reflection, the practitioner may come to see the world differently...' The ability to reflect on evidence, and more importantly to reflect critically, has become an essential skill for the clinician of the future (Pietroni, 1998). For me, the research achieved its overall aim. The most encouraging finding was how strongly the student nurses felt about taking clinical supervision forward into their new roles. However, there is concern about the impact of student numbers, which appeared to be discouraging some of the universities from incorporating clinical supervision into pre-registration curricula. At the time I worked in partnership with the university to develop ways in which to introduce the process of supervision throughout the diploma curriculum.

There is still work to be undertaken but the importance of reflective practice and clinical supervision is obvious and there is a need for it to be incorporated within the pre-registration curriculum. The research needs to be continued because nurses and health professionals should feel valued and supported so that they can be responsive to the public's health care needs and also the health care economy.

References

Ajiboye P (2000) Learning partners. *Nursing Standard* **14**(51): 53

Antonsson A, Sandstroem B (2000) Reflection – The core in clinical supervision. *Vard I Norden Nursing Science and Research in the Nordic Countries* **20**(4): 38–41

Blaxter L (1996) *How to Research*. Buckingham, Open University Press

Blaxter L, Hughes C, Tight M (2002) *How to Research*. Buckingham, Open University Press

Bishop V (1994) Clinical supervision. *Nursing Times* **90**(48): 40–2

Bishop V (1998) Clinical supervision: What is going on? Results of a questionnaire. *Nursing Times Research* **3**(2): 141–50

Bright B (1995) What is 'reflective practice'? *Curriculum Hull* **16**(2): 69–88

Burns N, Grove S (2003) *Understanding Nursing Research*. Pennsylvania, Saunders

Butterworth T (1997) *It is good to talk*. School of Nursing Studies, University of Manchester

Butterworth T, Carson J, White E, Jeacock J, Clements A, Bishop V (1996) First steps towards evaluating supervision in nursing and health visiting. 1. Theory, policy and practice development: A review. *J Clin Nurs* **5**: 127–32

Cairns J (1998) Clinical supervision and the practice nurse. *J Community Nurs* **12**(9): 20–4

Cormack D (2002) *The Research Process in Nursing*. Oxford, Blackwell Science

Department of Health (1999) *Making a Difference*. London, HMSO

Department of Health (2000) *National Health Service Plan*. London, Department of Health

Donaldson L (2001) Safe high quality health care: Investing in tomorrow's leaders. *Quality in Health Care* **10**(Suppl 2): ii8–12

Dunn L (1999) Reap the benefits of clinical supervision. *Practice Nurse* **18**: 19–23

Durrai W, Kendrick K (1999) Implementing clinical supervision. *Prof Nurse* **14**(12): 849–52

Fisher M (1996) Using reflective practice in clinical supervision. *Prof Nurse* **11**(7): 443–5

Goorapah D (1997) Clinical supervision. *J Clin Nurs* **6**: 173–8

Hawkins P, Shohet R (1989) *Supervision in Helping Professions*. Buckingham, Open University Press

Inskipp F, Proctor B (1993) *Making the Most of Supervision: Professional Development for Counsellors and Trainees*. London, Cascade

Johns C, Freshwater D (1998) *Transforming Nursing through Reflective Practice*. Oxford, Blackwell Science

Jones A (1996) Orem's self-care model of clinical supervision. *Int J Palliat Nurs* **2**(2): 77–83

Jones A (1999) Clinical supervision for professional practice. *Nursing Standard* **14**(9): 42–4

Kok J, Chabeli MM (2002) Reflective journal writing: How it promotes reflective thinking in clinical nursing education: A students' perspective. *Curationis SA J Nurs* **25**(3): 35–42

Lepp M, Zorn CR, Duffy PR, Dickson RJ (2003) International education and reflection: Transition of Swedish and American nursing students to authenticity. *J Prof Nurs* **19**(3): 164–72

Lowry M (1998) Clinical supervision for the development of nursing practice. *Br J Nurs* **7**(9): 553–8

Marrow CE, Yaseen T, Cook M (1998) Caring together: Clinical supervision. RCN Nursing Update, *Nursing Standard* **12**: 22

May L (2003) Support systems. *Nursing Standard* **17**(24): 60–2

Murray K (2001) Overstretched lecturers say students are suffering. *Nursing Standard* **16**(10): 9

Myrick F (2002) Preceptorship and critical thinking in nursing education. *J Nurs Edu* **41**(4): 154–68

Nicklin P (1995) Super supervision. *Nurs Manag* **2**(5): 24–5

Nursing and Midwifery Council (2002) *Supporting Nurses and Midwives Through Lifelong Learning*. London, Nursing and Midwifery Council

Pietroni P (1998) Foreword. In Clarke R, Croft P (eds) *Critical Reading for the Reflective Practitioner*. Oxford, Butterworth-Heinemann

Price A, Chalker M (2000) Our journey with clinical supervision in an intensive care unit. *Intensive and Critical Care Nursing* **16**: 51–5

Pursey A (1995) Clinical supervision - A threat or an opportunity? *Nursing Times* **5**(3): 3

Robson C (2002) *Real World Research*. Boston, Blackwell Publishing

Rowan P, Barber P (2000) Clinical facilitators: A new way of working. *Nursing Standard* **14**(52): 35–8

Scanlon C, Weir W (1997) Learning from practice? Mental health nurses' perceptions and experiences of clinical supervision. *J Adv Nurs* **26**: 295–303

Schön D (1987) *Educating the Reflective Practitioner Towards a New Design for*

Teaching and Learning in the Professions. San Francisco, Jossey Bass

Severinsson E, Borgenhammar E (1997). Expert views on clinical supervision: A study based on interviews. *J Nurs Manag* **5**: 175–83

United Kingdom Central Council (1996) *Policy Statement on Clinical Supervision for Nursing and Health Visitors.* London, UKCC

Vaughan B (1996) Developing nursing. *Nursing Standard* **10**(15): 32–5

Webb B (1997) Auditing a clinical supervision training programme. *Nursing Standard* **11**(34): 34–9

Williams B (2001) *Developing Critical Reflection for Professional Practice Through Problem-Based Learning.* Williston, VT, Blackwell Science

CHAPTER 5

Action-learning sets and their place in clinical supervision

Sue Lillyman

Introduction

It needs to be emphasised that action-learning sets are not an additional process that professionals have to be involved in, but rather they can be part of the clinical supervision framework. They are an alternative to group clinical supervision consisting of a slightly different format. Action-learning sets, like clinical supervision, can help to fulfil the clinical governance agenda, provide evidence for the knowledge and skills framework (Department of Health, 2004), and help the practitioner achieve continual professional development requirements. They may involve any practitioner working at operational or strategic level within the organisation.

There are a lot of similarities between action-learning sets and group supervision and it is the intention of this chapter to clarify and gain an understanding of action-learning sets. I have used action-learning sets with a multidisciplinary team and those working at strategic levels within organisations and both have worked well. Douglas (2006) also noted their use in project management within a multidisciplinary team approach to collaborative working. However this has not been so successful with newly qualified staff nurses mainly due to the practitioners not having the skills to ask the challenging questions required for this approach. In this time of great change in the NHS, action-learning sets can help the practitioner keep up and manage that change. As Revans (1998) stated, learning must be equal to or greater than the rate of change.

What is action learning?

Although relatively new to nursing, action-learning sets were introduced into management education and development in 1975 (Pedler *et al*, 2005), with Revans has been identified as the 'father' of action learning (Marsick and O'Neil, 1999).

Pedler notes that there has been some controversy over the process because of it championing the ideas of practitioners or action learners over those of experts and teachers. Pedler (2005) goes onto remind us that the prime purpose of action learning is to do better things in the world and that action learning includes self-development in the context of action on urgent and intractable social problems. It was Revans who stated that 'all learning is for the sake of action and all action for the sake of friendship' (Revans, 1998: vii). Action learning is an approach to the development of people in organisations, which takes the task as the vehicle for learning. It is based on the premise that there is no learning without action and no sober and deliberate action without learning (Pedler, 1997).

What is an action-learning set?

If action learning is an approach to learning then action-learning sets are the framework that enables and supports that process to happen. Having been introduced into management in the 1970s action-learning sets were introduced into health care mainly through the Royal College of Nursing Clinical Leadership course (Royal College of Nursing, 2002). The Royal College of Nursing stated that an action-learning set consists of a group of individuals who are motivated and work together over an extended period of time. They are involved with peer supervision, reflecting on work-related experiences to develop an action plan that they then carry out in practice prior to the next meeting.

The set is made up of six to eight professionals; these can be peer groups or made up of a group of multiprofessionals working at any level within the organisation.

In the same way as group clinical supervision the set meets on a regular basis for an agreed amount of time out of practice. The meetings are normally held away from the place of work in an environment where the practitioners feel free to engage and share concerns. A facilitator is usually present to guide the process and assist the practitioners to listen, question, challenge and help form action plans for future work. The process is based on action from the reflection and shifts the centre of gravity from thought to action on the basis of learning.

According to the Royal College of Nursing (2002) there are three levels of learning that can be incorporated into an action-learning set. These can be about self, about an issue to be tackled and about the process of learning itself.

Principles of an action-learning set

The concept of an action-learning set is to provide a situation where practitioners feel safe to disclose their practice, gain support from colleagues and challenge each other in a supportive manner. They formulate action plans based on the discussions and reflections within the group that they then take back into practice. Following implementation of the action plan practitioners report back to the group the outcomes of their actions at the beginning of the next meeting.

Empathetic listening by group members is the key role during the process and time must be given for the person presenting the issue or concern to tell his or her story without interruption. After the presenter has shared the issue or concern the group and/or facilitator may ask questions for clarification and summarising. It is only when the group members feel that they have the story clear that open challenging questions may be asked. The group is expected to question using only open questions and not offer advice or solutions. This will assist the presenter to explore the issues raised for him or herself. The framework for these questions can be seen later in the chapter. The presenter is allowed time for critical reflection and feedback to the group. Once the questioning is complete the presenter uses the reflection to formulate a possible solution/action plan. Here it is suggested that critical reflection is engaged to explore the issue in the social context as well as reviewing individual concerns. The questioning element of the process is for clarification, to assist reflection and help practitioners develop their own action plan but not to challenge the presenters in such a way that they feel embarrassed or vulnerable.

Feedback is only given in order to clarify and summarise the issues and presenting practitioners will be expected to develop their own action plan from the questioning and challenges of the group.

In summary the group is there to support and challenge through:

* listening
* reflecting
* questioning
* giving feedback (Royal College of Nursing, 2002).

The main aims of the group members are to avoid imposing values and opinions, giving advice, being judgemental, criticising or trivialising. The process allows individuals to learn from experience, share experience, have colleagues' challenge and support, take the challenge and implement it, and review with colleagues the action taken and lessons learnt (Revans, 1998). Pedler (1991) states that there are three components of these sets including: people who accept the responsibility for taking action on a particular issue; problems or tasks that people set themselves; and a set of six or so colleagues who support and challenge each other to make progress on problems.

Who can be part of the action-learning set?

As stated earlier anybody can be a member of an action-learning set, however all participants should join voluntarily, be committed to the process and have some understanding of how the action-learning set works. This approach has worked well within a multiprofessional team as well as with a mixture of staff from all disciplines, both clinical and non-clinical, coming together to talk through issues that relate to their practice. The group uses the process to develop an action plan in order to celebrate, change or adapt their practice. Practitioners need to have a common concern for improving practice.

Benefits of the action-learning set

The Royal College of Nursing (2002) stated that professionals who take part in an action-learning set have noted an increase in confidence and self-awareness. They reported that they were able to approach situations from a broader and more political perspective. They feel that through the process they are more proactive than reactive and reflective rather than emotional. Participants feel that they have developed listening skills and are achieving their goals faster than expected. They reported that they are able to develop and stimulate others in the organisation.

The group learns from experience and shares that experience where colleagues can support and challenge each other. Critical reflection forms an integral part of the process and allows the practitioner to review the action taken and the consequences of that action and identify lessons learnt. As Mezirow (1991) suggested critical reflection is powerful as it encourages a transformation of perspectives. However, Weinstein (1995) notes that this can be disturbing for those who do not want to change their practice and the facilitator must be aware of this.

Setting up an action-learning set

As with group clinical supervision team members need to be committed to the process and set their own ground rules for the meetings. The ground rules should include confidentiality, respect for other group members, commitment to the process, turning off of mobile phones, time keeping, participation in group discussion and so on. Often it is useful to have a facilitator to act as the timekeeper and to prevent the group offering advice or judgements. Facilitators also make sure groups use appropriate and open challenging questions to help presenters develop their own action plans. If a facilitator is used he or she does not contribute to the reflective process (Royal College of Nursing, 2002).

The first session will normally involve the facilitator identifying how the process works and some of the models that can be employed within the action-learning set to discuss the issues raised. The group should ideally meet away from the work area and on a monthly basis. The meetings may last between one and two hours depending on the availability of the group members and this should be agreed before the group starts. Individual members of the group share an issue;

this can be an area of good practice that they wish to celebrate or an area of concern. The other members do not participate at this stage but allow room for the presenters to tell their story. Following the presentation the group members can use questions to clarify issues. Each member will require at least half an hour to explore his or her issue and therefore all the group members might not be able to share in each meeting. There should be a rota to ensure each group member has the opportunity to share an issue of concern over a set amount of months. However all members are expected to participate with the questioning. Once the presenter has clarified the issue for the group then the group can use open challenging questions. This questioning should not be judgemental, nor should group members give their own opinions or trivialise the situation. These questions help presenters to reflect critically, to learn from that practice and formulate their own action plans that they will implement prior to the next meeting.

At the start of subsequent meetings there should be an opportunity for an update from participants to feed back on the implementation of their plans so that the group can discuss and learn for their own professional development. The group may use a variety of different models to accommodate people's different approaches to learning as discussed below. The discussion needs to focus on an in depth problem solving critical reflection as stated earlier.

Isaacs (1999) sums this up by identifying four requirements for dialogue: listening, respecting, suspending and voicing.

The role of the facilitator

Facilitators are skilled practitioners who provide an understanding of the nature of professional practice through the provision of learning opportunities and supportive intervention (Morton-Cooper and Palmer, 1993), and who have a commitment to ongoing education (Armitage and Burnard, 1991). Their role is to keep time and oversee the process in the form of the questions asked within the group and uphold the ground rules set by the group. They encourage the group to participate in the action-learning set and can bounce questions back to the group for clarification as well as challenge the group. The role is that of encourager, helping to identify problems and form action plans. They help the group to summarise and seek clarification, highlighting any key issues raised within the discussion and provide feedback to the group helping group members to expand the vision. Their main roles are summarised by the Royal College of Nursing (2002) as questioning to clarify, confirming and challenging.

Group clinical supervision or action-learning set?

Although group clinical supervision and action-learning sets are similar there are some fundamental differences that need to be addressed:

Similarities

- Both approaches, as stated previously, help towards meeting the clinical governance agenda and the individual's knowledge and skills framework (Department of Health, 2004).
- Both involve a set time out of practice to share with other professionals. The time frames are comparable and usually involve a monthly meeting consisting of one to two hours.
- Both groups involve critical reflection on issues presented to the group.
- With the reflection both help the participants learn from practice and identify areas for development and change.
- Both can be multidisciplinary in their approach and both benefit from a mixed group where sometimes aspects can be reviewed from different perspectives, ie. leadership or managerial issues.
- Both processes have a supervisor or facilitator who oversees the process.
- For the organisation, both may appear costly as they take the practitioner away from their area of work. However both have been evaluated and demonstrate an increase in quality of client care, reduced sickness and improved support for the participants.

Differences

- Group clinical supervision often includes a supervisor who is often more experienced than the participants and may guide the participants towards group discussion that leads to a group action plan. Action-learning sets have a facilitator who is not involved in the questioning but is there to keep time and to challenge and support the process based on a model of questioning.
- Clinical supervision may include sharing of ideas and opinions in order to assist the presenter to reach a plan of action whereas the action-learning set only uses challenging open questions that allow the presenter to work out his or her own action plan.
- Although both include reflection as part of the process the action-learning set uses critical reflection to explore social issues around the problem being addressed. Clinical supervision focuses more on individuals and their immediate problems and/or concerns.
- Both approaches use models. Clinical supervision tends to use those described in *Chapter 1,* for example, Proctor's (1992) three function interactive model, Faugier's (1992) growth and support model, or Hawkins and Shohet's (1998) integrative approach. Action-learning sets are based on the work of Rogers (1969) and take a person-centred, unconditional positive regard approach.

- Action-learning sets are more about the involvement of group participants rather than group dynamics (Revans, 1998) which is often seen in clinical supervision.

Techniques for questioning in action-learning sets

Group members should be given the choice of technique they wish to use within the action-learning set and this should be the one they feel most comfortable with. The techniques suggested by the Royal College of Nursing (2002) in their facilitators' toolkit include: De Bono's six thinking hats, six shoes and six medals approaches; Kipling's six honest serving men; strengths, weaknesses, opportunities and threats (SWOT) analysis; force field analysis; role set analysis; perceptual positions; the three brains; mind mapping; appreciative inquiry; brain storming or shower thoughts; issues and feelings; jumping in with both feet; concept analysis; Z-technique; circle of concern and circle of influence; and integrative approach.

Some of these are discussed below.

Six thinking hats

De Bono (2004) used the six thinking hats approach to help sort out people's thoughts and focus on one aspect of a situation. The six hats all have different colours and each represents a different mode. When wearing a hat the person can only use that particular approach, ie.

- The black hat is concerned with critical thinking; it allows us to judge what is right or wrong. We can see if it fits our own values, resources, strategies and ability. It also allows for moans and gripes.
- The white hat indicates neutrality and is used to collect the facts together. No opinions or interpretations are used when wearing this hat. It helps review what we know, what we need to know, what is missing, what we should ask, and how we might get the information we need. It is concerned with soft personal information.
- The red hat represents fire and warmth, our emotions, feelings and intuitions.
- The yellow hat is about positive thinking and beginning constructive and positive assessment. It helps us to review our values and benefits and questions why something should work. While wearing this hat De Bono notes that insights might happen.
- The green hat is for creative thinking, a need to explore beyond the known and obvious. It allows us to explore the alternatives.
- The blue hat is for control, summarising, overviews and conclusions.

The person presenting might use the hats or the group can use them when probing and challenging and helping the presenter to reflect.

Six shoes

De Bono's (1996) six shoe approach also uses different styles and colours of shoes but in a slightly different approach to the hats. This approach also helps the group choose a course of direction. Orange gumboots are used for urgent action to avert a crisis or deal with an emergency situation, pink slippers are used for caring or helping, and navy formal shoes are for authority, rules or regulations to be adhered to. Brown sensible shoes are for practice action, purple riding boots for extraordinary action and grey sneakers for investigation and collection of information.

Six value medals

The six value medals were described by De Bono in 2005. Here he uses six medals to denote different values.

- Gold: human values.
- Silver: organisational values associated with money.
- Steel: quality issues and strength.
- Glass: innovation, simplicity and creativity.
- Wood: environmental concerns.
- Brass: perceptual values.

Each colour is related to the value being explored and focuses the discussion.

Six honest serving men

This approach is based on the poem by Rudyard Kipling and is useful as an aid memoir for phrasing questions. The poem goes:

I had six honest serving men
(They taught me all I knew)
Their names where What and Why and When
And How and Where and Who.

Kipling (1960: 60).

To include this in the action-learning set the group asks open questions based on the philosophy of the poem. This prevents the giving of opinions and focuses the group on open-ended questions in order to explore the issue being discussed.

SWOT analysis

SWOT is where people question and review each aspect of an issue (Rogers, 1999). They review each aspect in relation to themselves, their professional practice and the organisational constraints and commitments. Completing the analysis often helps the person see things from another point of view.

Force field analysis

Lewin (1963) developed force field analysis. This is where the driving forces are in conflict with the restraining forces causing an instability and a maintenance of the status quo of a situation. The latter are resistance to change. Group members are invited to brainstorm ideas for the forces at work and then analyse them to determine the needs and priorities to be addressed in planning for change through strengthening the forces. Changing the direction of a force, withdrawing forces or adding new helping forces helps to identify the action plan.

Mind mapping

The concept of mind mapping has been outlined in Ghaye and Lillyman (2006) where mind mapping was used in a learning journal. Three elements or nodes were used to represent key ideas with linking lines being drawn between the nodes. These lines revealed relationships and gave meaning to the nodes by nature of the links between them. Group members are encouraged to draw on a flip chart their thought processes and use them to clarify the connections with challenging questions.

This approach may help focus on the issues and might help to fine-tune 'know what' and 'know why' knowledge, or change the perception of aspects being discussed.

Perceptual positioning

Perceptual positioning is described by the Royal College of Nursing (1996) and is used to gain insight into one's own behaviour and that of others. It consists of three positions: The first is in your own reality, which includes the aspect being presented, and seeing and feeling reality in that role. Failing to move from this position could leave the person with the same issues and may lead to a lack of insight or what Johari states as exploring the blind self (see *Chapter 1*). The second position is stepping out of the self and taking someone else's point of view. Looking into the situation might give another insight; it might open up a blind window as another view is taken. The third position is what is referred to as the fly on the wall and the ability to step back out of the situation and view it from a totally different perspective, ie. see the issue from the outside.

Z-technique

This helps if the group begins to lose its way and needs to refocus. It is based on Myers Briggs' Type Indicator (Rogers 1999) and includes four key questions:

- What are the facts/data?
- What are the possibilities?
- What are the logical implications of any choice made?
- What is the likely impact on people of any of the choices?

The five whys

This focuses on the root of the problem (Senge *et al*, 1994). The question 'Why did this happen?' is asked. Answers are explored and the question 'Why?' is asked of the answer. This is repeated up to five times for subsequent answers and assists the presenter to explore thoroughly the underlying values and assumptions made and gain a deeper reflection into the issue being addressed.

Summary

As Van Zwanenberg and Harris (2000) state we can look at the glass or we can look through it to see the bigger picture. The techniques identified above help the group to look through and beyond the immediate issues. The action learning process focuses on empathetic listening, challenging supportive questioning and feedback. This approach can be used in place of group clinical supervision and can be used as part of the clinical governance agenda with written reflections and action plans as evidence for the Knowedge and Skills Framework and professional body requirements for the practitioner.

References

Armitage P, Burnard P (1991) Mentors or preceptors? Narrowing the theory practice gap. *Nurse Education Today* **11**: 225–9

De Bono E (1996) *Six Action Shoes*. London, Harper Collins

De Bono E (2004) *How to Have a Beautiful Mind*. London, Vermillion

De Bono E (2005) *The Six Value Medals*. London, Vermillion

Department of Health (2004) *The NHS Knowledge and Skills Framework and Development Review Process*. London, Department of Health

Douglas S (2006) A model for setting up interdisciplinary collaborative working in groups: Lessons from an experience of action learning. *J Psych Ment Health Nurs* **11**(2): 189–93

Faugier J (1992) The supervisory relationship in clinical supervision and mentorship in nursing. In Butterworth T, Faugier J (eds). *Clinical Supervision and Mentorship in Nursing*. London, Chapman and Hall

Ghaye T, Lillyman S (2006) *Learning Journals and Critical Incidents. Reflective Practice for Health Care Professionals* (2nd edn). Dinton, Quay Books

Hawkins P, Shohet R (1989) *Supervision in the Helping Professions*. Milton Keynes, Open University Press

Isaacs W (1999) *Dialogue and the Art of Thinking Together*. New York, Doubleday

Kipling R (1960) *Just So Stories*. London, Purnell Books

Lewin K (1963) *Field Theory in Social Science: Selected Theoretical Papers*. London, Tavistock

Marsick V, O'Niel J (1999) The many faces of action learning management learning. *J Manag Organizational Learning* **2**: 159–76

Mezirow J (1991) *Transforming Dimensions of Adult Learning*. San Francisco, Jossey Bass

Morton-Cooper A, Palmer A (1993) *Mentoring and Preceptorship*. Oxford, Blackwell Scientific

Pedler M (ed) (1991) *Action Learning in Practice* (2nd edn). Brookfield VT, Gower

Pedler M (ed) (1997) *Action learning in Practice* (3rd edn). Aldershot, Gower

Pedler M (2005) Editorial. *Action Learning Research and Practice* **2**(1): 1–6

Pedler M, Burgoyne J, Brook C (2005) What has action learning learned to become? *Action Learning Research and Practice* **2**(1): 49–68

Proctor B (1992) *Supervision in the Helping Professions*. Milton Keynes, Open University Press

Revans RW (1992) *The Origins and Growth of Action Learning*. Bromley, Cartwell Bratt

Revans RW (1998) *ABC of Action Learning*. London, Lemos and Crane

Rogers C (1969) *Freedom to Learn*. Ohio, Merrill

Rogers J (1999) *Facilitating Groups*. London, Management Futures

Royal College of Nursing (1996) *Nursing Leadership – Study Guide*. London, Royal College of Nursing

Royal College of Nursing (2002) *Facilitators Toolkit: Techniques for Action Learning Sets*. RCN Clinical Leadership Team. London, Royal College of Nursing

Senge P, Kleiner A, Roberts C, Ross RX, Smith B (1994) *The Fifth Discipline Field Book: Strategies and Tools for Building a Learning Organization.* London, Nicholas Brealey

Van Zwanenberg T, Harrison J (2000) *Clinical Governance in Primary Care.* Oxford, Radcliffe Medical Press

Weinstein K (1995) *Action Learning: A Journey in Discovery and Development.* London, Harper Collins

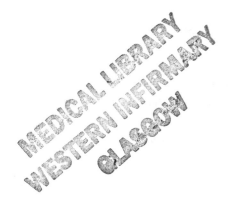

CHAPTER 6

Clinical supervision as experience-based improvement

Tony Ghaye

In the Nursing and Midwifery Council's (NMC) publication, *Supporting Nurses and Midwives Through Lifelong Learning* (2004: 7) there is a definition of clinical supervision. It reads:

Clinical supervision aims to bring practitioners and skilled supervisors together to reflect on practice, to identify solutions to problems, to increase understanding of professional issues and, most importantly, to improve standards of care.

This important statement is worth a closer look.

- *Who is involved?* Answer: practitioners and skilled supervisors. How far does this sound like two kinds of people to you?
- *What do they do?* Answer: they identify solutions to problems, increase understanding of professional issues and improve standards of care. How far is this appropriate? In this trilogy, what dominates? Is it the bringing and the solving of problems?
- *How do they identify, understand and improve?* Answer: through reflection on practice. So what kinds of reflective practices might a skilled supervisor enable a practitioner to engage with in order to achieve one or more of these things?

The rhetoric

In 2006 the NMC issued this statement in their advice sheets:

Clinical supervision should be available to registrants throughout their careers so they can constantly evaluate and improve their contribution to patient/ client care. Along with the NMC's PREP [continuing professional development] standard, clinical supervision is an important part of clinical governance... The

NMC supports the principle of clinical supervision but believes that it is best developed at a local level in accordance with local needs. We do not, therefore, advocate any particular model of clinical supervision and we do not provide detailed guidance about its nature and scope. Instead, the NMC has defined a set of principles, which we believe should underpin any system of clinical supervision that is used.

The principles are:

- Clinical supervision supports practice, enabling registrants to maintain and improve standards of care.
- Clinical supervision is a practice-focused professional relationship, involving a practitioner reflecting on practice guided by a skilled supervisor.
- Registrants and managers should develop the process of clinical supervision according to local circumstances. Ground rules should be agreed so that the supervisor and the registrant approach clinical supervision openly, confidently and are aware of what is involved.
- Every registrant should have access to clinical supervision and each supervisor should supervise a realistic number of practitioners.
- Preparation for supervisors should be flexible and sensitive to local circumstances. The principles and relevance of clinical supervision should be included in pre-registration and post-registration education programmes.
- Evaluation of clinical supervision is needed to assess how it influences care and practice standards. Evaluation systems should be determined locally.

Again let us have a close look at these principles. What do we learn?

- Clinical supervision is essentially about maintaining and improving standards of care.
- To achieve this we have to learn from our practice, with one person (a supervisee) being guided by another skilful person (a supervisor).
- The process works best when those involved feel they can be open and confident and are aware of what is involved.
- Supervisors should not be over-burdened with too many supervisees.
- Supervisors should be well prepared for their role.
- Clinical supervision needs evaluating to assess its impact on quality of care.

At the heart of all of this is a view that clinical supervision is essentially about the positive and practical use of experience derived from clinical practice. This experience could be personal or collective; about you, or you with others. Another way of putting this is that clinical supervision is a learning process. And because it is (largely) about learning from practice, it involves re-experiencing something (either alone with a supervisor, or within a supportive group) that is felt, and thought, to be significant in some way and worthy of talking about. However, the process is not all backward looking, or retrospective. Because of the emphasis on personal standards and on improving future care, it must also be forward looking, or prospective. If we wrap all this together we can come up with a statement of the kind 'clinical supervision is an experienced-based improvement process'. The NMC's statements represent what we might regard as policy. Some might say that it is rhetoric. In other words this is what the regulatory body for these two professions say it should be.

Some realities

So what about some (experienced) realities? In other words how does the rhetoric work out in practice? This will, of course, vary from place to place. Recent research by Davey *et al* (2006) describes a large-scale, naturally representative sample of nurses who qualified with a nursing diploma between 1997 and 1998. In their paper Davey *et al* present the experience of 1918 of these nurses in their early career, 18 months after qualification, from adult, child, learning disability and mental health branches. The article is about who gets something called clinical supervision in nursing. They ask the specific question, 'So what is it?', with the 'it' being clinical supervision. They came up with some interesting findings. For example, they say:

> *There is no single, clear definition of clinical supervision. There are however common themes, in particular the functions of developing skills and learning through a reflective process involving both a supervisor and supervisee.*
>
> (Davey *et al*, 2006: 239)

That there is no single and clear definition of clinical supervision perhaps reflects the fact that it is a 'broad church'. There are many views of it and many ways to practise it. Perhaps we should applaud this plurality. On the other hand how do we evaluate something if there is no clear definition of what it is?

Davey *et al* (2006) reported a significant variation of experience between nurses on each branch. They found that only 38% of their sample were receiving something called clinical supervision and of those who were, 35% never had a clinical supervisor. Perhaps this suggests that other kinds of 'facilitation' were in place, for example, co-supervision, some kind of peer support, or group supervision. In terms of 'getting assistance with reflection on practice' only 53–65% of nurses had their needs met. So how were more than 35% of nurses in the sample being enabled to learn from their practice? Additionally 68–74% of the sample had their needs met with regard to 'discussing incidents which occur at work'. This may not be as good as it might seem at first glance. So what were the other 25% discussing if it was not incidents that occurred at work? They reported that 40% of nurses in the child branch and 35% in the adult branch wanted more help with reflection on practice. So what does this say about the skilfulness of the supervisors? There were also substantial unmet needs in the sample (33–45%), in terms of the nurses receiving an 'evaluation of their performance'. So how can anyone set up their own personal improvement or learning agenda, if they do not have a full and balanced view of their strengths and growth points? Allied to this, 'receiving constructive feedback' was another marked unmet need reported by 23–43% of the sample.

Provocative questions

So where does this leave us? When forms of clinical supervision work well, they clearly serve a very useful purpose. But perhaps it is time to ask some tough questions. Clearly clinical supervision is a process experienced differently by those involved. Maybe this challenges the rather naïve assumption that it is good for everyone. Are the current views we have of clinical supervision the most appropriate? In its present forms, is it worth the investment? Is it sustainable given what is happening in the health 'system' as a whole? If clinical supervision is about improving standards of care, and not only about personal professional development, where is the evidence that directly links forms of clinical supervision with improvements in patient/client experiences? Is it at best a curate's egg, at worst all a bit of a masquerade? By this I mean the rhetoric is one of liberation, enlightenment and empowerment.

In reality, if we were only able to acknowledge it, clinical supervision may simply be a clever form of institutional surveillance. This surveillance is operationalised through the skilled supervisor who acts in a cloak of performance monitoring. 'They' monitor what 'we' do. On the face of things, skilled supervisors offer support and advice. But in reality their skilfulness is a form of covert control. Their role is really one of stabilising the dominant discourses and practices. It is not about professional growth but about control and reinforcing the status quo. Could it be possible that clinical supervision has been sabotaged by routinisation, that all we have done is turn something which could potentially be very helpful, into yet another NHS 'model' that can be applied as a veneer to satisfy the agendas of practice development/ educators and professional politicists? Arguably a central problem is that clinical supervision never gets sufficiently embedded and internalised within healthcare organisations to disturb the dominant discourses and ways of doing things. In other words it is a kind of 'clinical ceremonial'. Clinical supervision is not a form of constructive resistance, a celebration of difference and the possibility that things can be otherwise. It is not a force for anything other than (at best) reframing individual practices. So all we get are pockets or islands of enlightened and more insightful practitioners with the courage to improve care, locally. But is this enough?

In reality, to be able to talk about clinical supervision is to add a sense of gravitas to professional development, a process that may normally be fragile, interrupted, incompatible with 'the way things are done around here', and messy. But does this sense of gravitas simply seek to quieten those colleagues who believe clinical supervision is about 'the confessional', the touchy-feely, the luxury activity and the frivolous?

Clinical supervision as a lived experience

One of the NMC's principles is that experiencing clinical supervision is predicated upon the setting of ground rules 'so that the supervisor and the registrant approach clinical supervision openly, confidently and are aware of what is involved'. Again we need to take a careful look at the implications of this. Hyrkäs *et al* (2006) state that an array of things influence the quality of the supervisory experience. For example, the characteristics of the supervisors, how well the supervisors are trained to do the job, whether the supervisees actually chose their supervisors or whether they were allocated to them in some way, whether it is a one-to-one or small group experience, whether the supervisors are from the supervisees' own discipline or not, the supervisees' previous experiences of supervision and so on. Trust between both (or all) parties and individual expectations of the process, all affect the experience. Putting the NMC's principle under some pressure might reveal those aspects of the psychosocial 'context' of clinical supervision we need to think about.

Scenario 1: Things that would improve my experience of working here (the view of a qualified nurse)

What follows is part of a statement made by a nurse, in a one-to-one meeting with her supervisor. Imagine you are the supervisor here. Your supervisee discloses the following to you. This is how it all tumbled out at the beginning of one such meeting. How does it make you feel? What are you thinking about? What might you say to her?

> *It seems to me that we pretty much do the same things every day without any real change. It's worrying isn't it? We feel the same way, usually a bit fed up. We experience the same problems. We know what they are, but nothing seems to get done about them. So I've given some things some thought. I hope you don't mind. For example, I really think having a designated room for nursing staff to take their breaks would help so much. And I really need a better work station in which to do my paperwork. Having regular in-house training days and a reflective*

sessions twice weekly, rather than monthly, would be a good idea. We also need to operate as an effective team. We would benefit from team building exercises especially as our area is changing and we have a few new staff. Meeting with other staff (not nurses) to discuss cases and improving the relationship with some practitioners would be very valuable. I could go on but you said these meetings were about trying to improve care for our patients. I don't feel we can do this unless we look after ourselves better. Now that's all the positive stuff.

This next lot isn't [looking down at some scribbled notes on the back of an envelope] a moan, but I feel it is important if we are going to work better. Staff who repeatedly perform poorly, who refuse to take responsibility, who arrive late for work, are absent from shifts (ie. are unreliable) should be sacked, including staff who cannot organise their own childcare. Why should their more reliable colleagues be expected to prop up the service and be paid no more than those sitting at home on sick leave or carer's leave? For this reason I think the NHS is viewed as a weak employer that does not value its loyal employees and allows widespread waste of taxpayer's money by continuing to employ work-shy people. This really gets me. Anyway enough for now. So what do you think?

Scenario 2: Improving my experience of this service (the view of a 32-year-old British woman having her second baby)

In the previous scenario, the 'experience' comes from a member of staff. The owner of it is present in the room. This is the raw material that forms the basis of a reflective conversation. In this scenario, the source of the experience is different. Here the reflective conversation in a small group clinical supervision meeting was fuelled by the presentation of a women's experience of childbirth. These data were gathered through a patient experience questionnaire called *Learning From You* (Institute of Reflective Practice UK, 2007). The experience was read out.

I requested some pain relief especially an epidural at 2cm, then 4cm but was refused. I was given some medication. There was no midwife present with me throughout my established labour and my partner and mum were furious with them. We were constantly asking them to help out, but to no avail. I was still on the ward at this point and only when I said I was going to push, was I rushed in a wheelchair to the labour room. My cervix was 9cm and my daughter was born one hour later. I had four different midwives coming in and out whilst pushing. The room was full of rubbish with someone else's placenta bits still left in the sink and a whole room full of rubbish sacks. It was filthy and not fit for a newborn to enter the world. I hemorrhaged and had four units of blood. My experience was of total neglect during labour and I am very upset that this bad management of midwives ruined my labour.

How does this make you feel? What are you thinking about? What might you say to others in the group? How does openness and confidentiality (embraced in the NMC principle cited above) work in these practical situations?

The importance of asking questions

Asking questions that matter can be a hard thing to do, because we are so used to thinking in terms of problems. Root causes of problems to be discovered, problems to be solved, things to be 'fixed'. Sometimes, creative and lasting improvements in care (a fundamental aim of clinical supervision) can begin when we start to ask questions, and to do this together. Asking questions marks the start of an experienced-based, learning conversation. This is a very different thing from many of our 'normal' conversations which often tend to be about problems. Here our talking and listening often fails to solve a problem because of the way that most of us talk and listen, most of the time. You may find it hard to accept, but our most common way of talking is telling; asserting this or that. Talking at the expense of asking. And our most common way of listening is not really listening at all. At best it is an impoverished view of listening, one where we only listen to our own voice, not to the voices of others. This has big implications for clinical supervision. If we are unable to talk openly about the complex problems (or challenges) that face us in our work, we get stuck. So what happens next? There are two ways to un-stick a conversation. The first is for one person or group to act unilaterally, to impose on others (no matter how well disguised) their solution to the problem. The 'supervisor knows best' syndrome. This is the playing out of the asymmetrical power dynamics inherent in the supervisor–supervisee relationship. Another way to get unstuck is to ask a question.

The power of the positive question

There are many kinds of question that are useful in a clinical supervision meeting. The two most common are open and closed questions. An open question is an invitation to express a point of view. A closed one usually invites a 'yes' or 'no' response. Another kind of question is a genuine one for which we do not already have answers. These questions are an invitation to be creative. They invite new ideas and insight. For example, the following experience was presented in a peer group (clinical supervision) meeting. In summary, two district nurses were visiting an elderly lady who had fallen while out shopping. She had twisted her ankle badly and bumped her head. The elderly lady could not remember much about the incident. One of the nurses suggested to the lady that she stayed at home, rested her leg and did not think of going to the shops again for a while. The lady became visibly distressed. She enjoyed going to the shops. She wanted to visit the town library, her friends and go to church. The other nurse said,

'What would happen if we thought about this differently?' This carefully framed question, genuine and sincere, invited a new way of understanding the lady's situation. It invited a new and different conversation. Carefully framed questions can develop a climate of openness in supervision sessions.

We might also use positive questions. If we focus and start to inquire into our problems, we begin to construct a world in which problems are central. They become the dominant realities that burden us every day. To ask questions about our failings is to create a world in which failing is focal. Deficit-based questions lead to deficit-based conversations, which in turn lead to deficit-based patterns of action. Yet we can flip this over and apply the same logic more positively. By asking ourselves positive questions we may bring forth future action of far greater promise. Positive questions invite positive action. So the 'climate' in a supervision session is linked to the kinds of questions we are asking. My suggestion is that we try to ask questions that get those involved to focus on what is positive and good about the situation being discussed, no matter in how small in amount. This can be followed up by seeking ways to amplify the positive because it is the positive that we want more of. If we focus our reflective conversations on problems, we are simply putting all our energy into trying to get rid of something. So where would you want to put your energy? With these thoughts in mind, what are the positive aspects within each of the two scenarios above?

Trust as a prerequisite for experienced-based improvement through clinical supervision

The importance of trust for both personal and team improvement has been discussed elsewhere (Ghaye, 2005). Although a complex process to establish and sustain, trust is usually assumed to be a prerequisite for building shared values, meanings and positive action. Trust is not always easy to achieve, especially where the weight of past betrayals and hostility hangs heavy (Rothstein, 2000).

Without trust, reflective conversations of positive regard are non-starters. Reina and Reina (2006) help us with two things: to appreciate how important trust (and betrayal) are in the workplace and how to build trusting relationships. At the heart of their book is the notion of transactional trust. This is a process of mutual exchange, reciprocity and something created incrementally over time. In other words we have to trust in order to increase the likelihood that we will be trusted. Reina and Reina set out three types of transactional trust:

■ *Contractual trust:* This is essentially a trust of character. Put another way, it is people actually doing what they promise they will do. It is about keeping agreements, honouring intentions and behaving consistently.

- *Communication trust:* This is essentially a trust of disclosure. Put another way, it is about people's willingness to share information, to tell the truth, admit mistakes, celebrate achievements and successes, maintain confidentiality, and give and receive constructive feedback. Trust influences the quality of our conversations and vice versa. This kind of trust underpins the stated value of a patient-led NHS.
- *Competence trust:* This is essentially a trust of capability. How far do you trust the people in your supervision group or trust the people you hand over to? Do you trust them to do a good job? How capable do you feel your colleagues are in giving you constructive feedback? How capable are they in providing you with what you think you want and need to know, in order to continue to improve your practice?

The experience of clinical supervision is heightened when we think deeply about two fundamental questions, 'What do I believe about others?' and 'What can I learn from others?'

Experienced-based improvement through open listening

Kahane (2004) gives us a sharp reminder of how not to conduct ourselves when we have the opportunity to have improvement-focused conversations. He says:

> The root of not listening is knowing. If I already know the truth, why do I need to listen to you? Perhaps out of politeness or guile I should pretend to listen, but what I really need to do is to tell you what I know, and if you don't listen, to tell you again, more forcefully. All authoritarian systems rest on the assumption that the boss can and does know the one right answer.
>
> (Kahane, 2004: 47).

Communication trust means talking openly and honestly. It brings with it a willingness and ability on our part to disclose to others what is in our head and heart. Listening openly, on the other hand, means being willing and able to positively embrace something different and new from others. This is not as easy as it may sound because it involves issues about interpersonal relations, power, value alignment and so on.

> My team worked hard to learn how to listen, without judging to what another person was trying to say – really to be there. If we listen in the normal closed way, for what is right and what is wrong, then we won't be able to hear what is possible ... We won't be able to create anything new.
>
> (Kahane, 2004, p. 77).

Listening sounds simple doesn't it? So when was the last time you felt you were listened to openly? How far can you think of a positive experience between you and a colleague when you felt you were listening openly? How do you know this? What made you feel this way? What were the circumstances that led up to this? What was the root cause of such a positive experience?

What kinds of behaviours support the way we might listen openly to and learn from colleagues in a clinical supervision meeting? How might this help us build a conversation between us of positive regard? Wheatley (2002: 28) offers us some useful thoughts in what she eloquently describes as 'seeing how wise we can be together'. What we can learn from her work is that we have not only to learn to listen openly, but also to listen reflectively. She recommends that:

- *We need to learn how to acknowledge one another as equals:* A language of positive regard requires us to acknowledge that we are equal as human beings (unequal when in role) and that we need each other. We cannot always improve our own practice and services by trying to figure things out on our own.

- *We should try to stay curious about each other:* We need to be genuinely interested in what our colleagues have to say, not fearful. We need to test out our commitment to a value of the kind, 'I believe that I can learn something significant from every colleague I meet, each day' (Ghaye and Lillyman, 2000). This weaves openness together with reflection.

- *We need to help each other listen openly and then act appropriately:* It can be hard work to listen, especially when we are busy, feeling certain of ourselves, or stressed. Try to think of a positive experience with your colleagues when you know you listened to their views and then acted appropriately on them? What made this a positive experience?

- *We need to slow down to make time to listen reflectively:* If listening is an important part in developing a language of positive regard, so too is slowing down. Often we need to make time to listen to each other's views and to reflect on them. A conversation in a supervision session should not be experienced as a rush through to the end of a list.

- *We should expect conversations to be messy at times:* Usually conversations do not move in a straight line. When learning in a supervision session, it is probable that some things do not appear to connect with our experiences and perceptions. Experiences can be diverse. Listening openly and reflectively means that we resist the impulse to tidy things up and put experiences in little boxes. We need to learn the benefits of being 'disturbed'. By this I mean having our ideas and practices challenged by others. How can we be creative in improving our own practice and improving health care services, if we are not willing to be disturbed?

To create new realities, we have to listen reflectively. It is not enough to be able to hear clearly the chorus of other voices; we must also hear the contribution of our own voice. It is not enough to be able to see others in the picture of what is going on; we must also see what we ourselves are doing. It is not enough to be observers of the problem situation; we must also recognise ourselves as actors who influence the outcome.

(Kahane, 2004: 83)

Your experience matters

Recently, in the context of service transformation, the NHS Institute for Innovation and Improvement has been talking about experience-based design. The process of clinical supervision as experienced-based improvement is constructively aligned with this. Experienced-based improvement is about improving ourselves, what we do, with whom and where, from a real understanding of our workplace experiences. Experienced-based improvement is an important outcome of clinical supervision where 'views' are shared and (hopefully) action taken. Improvement comes about by understanding the lived experiences (van Manen, 1997) of all those participating in the supervision meeting. How we feel affects how we think, which in turn affects what we (can) do.

Policing health care professionals

There has never been a more important time for some form of clinical supervision to be in place, in every healthcare organisation and available for all. The form of clinical supervision needs to achieve what it sets out to do and to be sustainable. The UK Government White Paper, *Trust, Assurance and Safety – The Regulation for Health Professionals in the 21st Century* (Department of Health, 2007) signals a major shake-up in the way health professions will be regulated. Staff will be regularly vetted on their competence and fitness to practise by their employer. Supervision, practice, learning and reflection are all mentioned in the White Paper, for example,

Excellence in education is the foundation of professional excellence in health care. The educational process takes individual potential and an individual sense of vocation and, through learning, practice, reflection, supervision, mentoring and examination, builds expertise, confidence and capability, and imbues students and trainees with a set of professional values and standards that they are expected to meet or exceed throughout their careers.

(Department of Health, 2007: 69).

Given this statement, the challenge is clear. Experienced-based improvement, through a process of clinical supervision, is a 'must happen' because it provides individuals with the necessary vocabulary, confidence and moral courage (Kidder, 2005) to explain and justify their practice in the new context of revalidation. If we fail to take up this challenge positively, the words of Virilio (1956: 66) 'today the surveillance screen tends to replace the window' may well be the lived reality for those in health care. Virilio's short sentence gives us much to reflect upon.

References:

Davey B, Desousa C, Robinson S, Murrells T (2006) The policy-practice divide – Who has clinical supervision in nursing? *J Res Nurs* **11**(3): 237–48

Department of Health (2007) *Trust, Assurance and Safety – The Regulation for Health Professionals in the 21st Century*. London, Stationary Office

Ghaye T (2005) *Developing the Reflective Healthcare Team*. Oxford, Blackwell Publishing

Ghaye T, Lillyman S (2000) *Reflection: Principles and Practice for Healthcare Professionals*. Wiltshire, Mark Allen Publishing

Hyrkäs K, Appelqvist-Schmidlechner K, Haataja R (2006) Efficacy of clinical supervision: Influence on job satisfaction, burnout and quality of care. *J Adv Nurs* **55**(4): 521–35

Institute of Reflective Practice UK (2007), *Learning From You*. Gloucester, Institute of Reflective Practice UK Publications

Kahane A (2004) *Solving Tough Problems*. San Francisco, Berrett-Koehler

Kidder R. (2005) *Moral Courage*. New York, HarperCollins

Nursing and Midwifery Council (2004) *Supporting Nurses and Midwives Through Lifelong Learning*. London, Nursing and Midwifery Council

Nursing and Midwifery Council (2006) *Advice Sheet: Clinical Supervision*. London, Nursing and Midwifery Council

Reina D, Reina M (2006) *Trust and Betrayal in the Workplace: Building Effective Relationships in Your Organization*. San Francisco, Berrett-Koehler

Rothstein B (2000), Trust, social dilemmas and collective memories. *Journal of Theoretical Politics* **4**: 477–501

van Manen M (1997) *Researching Lived Experience: Human Science for an Action Sensitive Pedagogy*. New York, SUNY Press

Virilio P (1956) *Cybermonde: La Politique du Pire*. Paris, Textual

Wheatley M (2002) *Turning to One Another: Simple Conversations to Restore Hope to the Future*. San Francisco, Berrett-Koehler Publishers

Index